SNAKES
& snake bite
in Southern Africa

Johan Marais

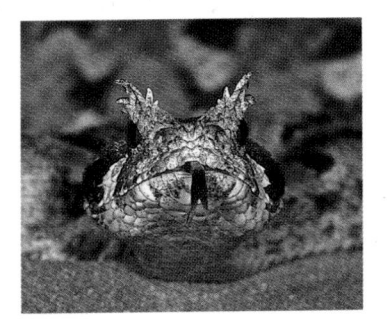

Struik Publishers (Pty) Ltd
(a member of The Struik New Holland Publishing Group (Pty) Ltd)
Cornelis Struik House
80 McKenzie Street
Cape Town 8001
Reg. No.: 54/00965/07

First published 1999

2 4 6 8 10 9 7 5 3 1

Publishing manager: Pippa Parker
Editor: Judy Bryant
Designer: Dominic Robson
Cover design: Danie Jansen van Vuuren

Reproduction by Disc Express, Cape (Pty) Ltd
Printed and bound by CTP (Pty) Ltd, Cape Town

Acknowledgments

During the last 20 or so years that I have had an active interest in herpetology, I have met
many amazing people; some incredibly talented, others very focused, and it has always been
a pleasure to spend time with them. We have had endless discussions, travelled together –
either photographing or looking for reptiles and amphibians – and these encounters have led
me to further interesting fields. Throughout this period I have had great support from a very
special friend, Donald Strydom, who has always supported me in every way possible. I am also
greatly indebted to Gerrie Smith, Paul Tan, Mac and Usha Madhav, Paul Moler and Randy Babb,
who have opened up my eyes to aspects of life I never considered. My thanks also go out to
Nush Goncalves, Brandon Borgelt, Timothy Simpkins, Dave Morgan, Theuns Eloff, Wulf Haacke,
Barry Stander, Mike Jaensch, Atherton de Villiers, Richard Boycott, Bill Branch, Gordon Setaro,
Lynn Raw, Mark Verseput and Mike Bates. Also to the long list of those whose names I have
not included. Marius Burger kindly supplied many of his excellent photographs. I have enjoyed
working with Pippa Parker of Struik Publishers and thank her for her patience.

Lastly, my sincere thanks to my family. My father has always fully supported me and
believed in me in everything that I have attempted. Molleen and Melissa, my wife and daugh-
ter, have always inspired and encouraged me. I spend a great deal of my time travelling and
working and, even when I am at home, they often only see glimpses of me as I come and go.
Their sacrifices, patience, love and support have given me the strength and perseverance not
to give up in life and face every day with enthusiasm, excitement and determination.

Johan Marais

CONTENTS

INTRODUCTION

Most people are afraid of snakes. Some are so terrified, they cannot even look at a picture of a snake or watch a documentary on snakes on television.

Snakes are in fact secretive creatures and most species will avoid humans at all costs, quickly slithering away when approached. When compared with mammals and birds, snakes may well be perceived to be somewhat strange. They have elongate, limbless bodies with extremely long backbones, and fragile ribs that are used for locomotion and to keep their bodies in shape. Furthermore, they lack eyelids and ears and have forked retractile tongues – incorrectly thought to harm or sting.

In many ways, snakes are far more effective than other predators. When a rodent disappears down its network of burrows, it is safe from most predators. But it is not out of reach of a snake, which can easily locate such prey within its burrow and may even devour its entire family in a single session.

Snakes as predators

Snakes are carnivores, many of them relying on muscle strength to overpower their prey, either swallowing it while it is half alive, or constricting it prior to swallowing. A snake first grabs onto its prey with its sharp teeth and then instantly throws a few coils around it. As the prey exhales, the snake tightens its coils until the victim succumbs to suffocation. It is a popular misconception that constrictors – the Southern African Rock Python for instance – crush their prey to death. In fact, no bones are broken when a snake constricts its prey.

Some snakes have evolved fangs and a venom apparatus designed for efficient capture of prey. This apparatus *may* be used in self-defence, but snake venoms are in fact quite slow to act in humans. Venoms are far more effective in killing prey, and also assist digestion. Certain venoms are prey-specific and are highly effective in killing certain prey species but have very little effect on others.

Snake venom is produced and stored in modified salivary glands which are situated in the upper jaw, more or less behind the eyes and at the side of the head. Saliva, one of the digestive juices secreted by animals, is particularly important to snakes as they cannot chew their food and have to swallow it whole.

If large food items are captured, snakes are able to dislocate their lower jaw, enabling them to swallow prey that is several times larger than the girth of the snake's own body.

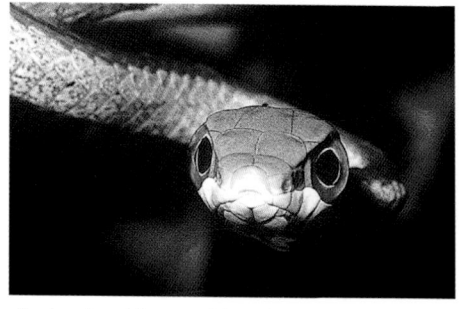

A Natal Bush Snake devours its reptile prey.

Vision

Despite popular belief, snakes are not able to hypnotise their prey. This misconception may have originated from the fact that snakes do not have eyelids and therefore cannot blink or cover their eyes. Snakes generally have good vision but tend to ignore stationary objects. A snake moving through the bush or among the branches of a tree can clearly see small objects and avoid them. In fact, in addition to scent, many snakes rely on detecting movement by sight so as to catch their prey. However, a snake chasing after a lizard or frog will momentarily lose sight of its prey if the latter freezes.

Snakes do not have eyelids and cannot blink or cover their eyes.

Snakes do not attack stationary objects, and this also applies to humans. People undertaking so-called 'snake sit-ins', enter cages with many venomous snakes. The moment one of the snakes get very close to the person, he or she merely freezes until the snake is at a safe distance again. Anyone coming across a snake, therefore, should freeze in their tracks. Under these circumstances, the snake will not approach closer to attack. Should the person choose to run away, however, the snake will not chase after them. Snakes *never* chase after people!

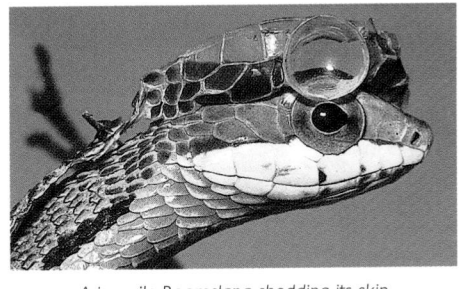

A juvenile Boomslang shedding its skin.

Hearing & smelling

Snakes have no external earholes and so cannot hear airborne sound. They are very sensitive to vibrations on the ground, however, and may sense the approach of a person on foot.

The somewhat 'sinister' forked tongue that one may see if closely observing a snake is completely harmless and cannot sting or harm in any way. It is used only for smelling. Snakes have unique organs situated in the roof of the mouth, known as the Organs of Jacobson. The ever-flicking tongue picks up particles in the air and deposits them onto the Organs of Jacobson, giving the snake a good idea of what is present in its immediate environment.

Snakes often inspect their dead prey with a flickering tongue prior to swallowing it. They do not lick their dead prey or cover it in saliva, however.

Growth & shedding

The external layer of a snake's skin does not grow; instead, the snake outgrows it and then sheds it. The entire layer of skin, from the tip of the nose to the tip of the tail, including the transparent caps that cover the eyes, is shed. In the wild, the skin is shed in one piece, much like an inverted sock, but in captivity, because conditions are not ideal, the skin usually comes off in pieces.

Prior to shedding, a snake's eyes become a pale blue colour; this condition is commonly described as the snake 'going into the blue'. When ready to shed, the snake will rub its nose on a stone or branch to loosen the old skin, then by crawling over a rough surface it will work the old skin off, exposing a healthy, often shiny, skin beneath it.

Snakes shed according to their growth rate and newly hatched snakes often shed for the first time within minutes of hatching. Juveniles may shed in excess of a dozen times in the first year and adults two or three times a year.

Reproduction

Mating among snakes occurs in spring, at which time females leave behind a scent trail that males follow with their flickering tongues. Several males may follow a single female. Once she is located, a mating ritual may follow, during which the male inspects the female – again with flickering tongue – perhaps even rubbing his chin up and down the sides of the female. Eventually he will twist the base of his tail beneath hers and copulation takes place.

Most snakes are egg-laying, or oviparous, depositing anything from two to 60 soft, leathery eggs at a time. The eggs may be laid in a hollow tree trunk, amongst decomposing vegetation, somewhere underground, or even in a deserted termite mound. It is important for the survival of the eggs that the female selects a laying site that is well protected from predators, such as monitor lizards or ants, and suitably damp to ensure that the eggs will not dry out before they hatch.

Most females deposit their eggs and move off, showing no further interest in them. Others, like some pythons, coil around the eggs and through muscular contractions that resemble hiccups, assist with the incubation process.

The young snakes that hatch from the eggs usually resemble the adults and have to fend for themselves immediately. Prior to leaving the eggs, the

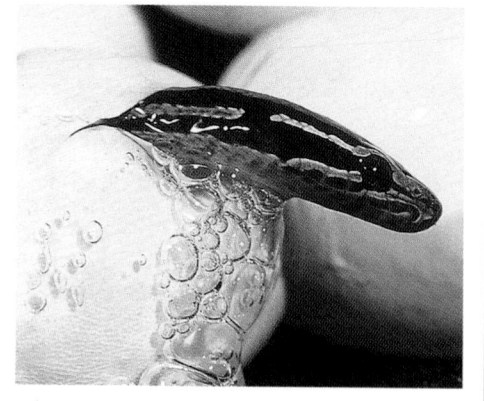

A newborn Brown House Snake cuts through its soft leathery eggshell.

young fill their abdomens with nutrient-rich yolk, which they can live off for several days. Hatchlings from venomous parents are also venomous from the moment they hatch and should never be regarded as harmless just because they are small.

Some snakes are viviparous, retaining the eggs within their bodies until they are ready to hatch, and seemingly giving birth to live young. The newborn young are covered in a fine membrane, from which they rupture free very soon after birth. Snakes from colder climates tend to be viviparous but in southern Africa there are no apparent reasons for some snakes laying eggs and others giving birth to live young. Mambas, cobras and pythons lay eggs while the Rinkhals, Mole Snake and most adders give birth to live young.

> The young of venomous snakes are themselves venomous from the moment they hatch. Small snakes should therefore not be handled as they could well be dangerous.

As a rule, snakes do not move around in pairs and if you come across a snake, it doesn't necessarily mean that it has a mate in the vicinity. Furthermore, snakes in our region do not have nests and newly hatched young soon move off in different directions to fend for themselves.

Body temperature & hibernation

Snakes, like all other reptiles, are cold-blooded or poikilothermic. This means that they have no internal mechanism to control their own body temperature and therefore have to rely on their immediate environment for their heat requirements.

Once it emerges from its overnight hideout, a snake may bask in the morning sun until its body temperature reaches an optimum level. It will then move about throughout the day, basking in the sun and alternately seeking shelter in order to maintain an acceptable level of body heat for it to function properly. After sunset, it may bask on a rock to benefit from absorbed heat before it retreats for the night. Many snakes bask on tarred roads at night for this reason and are then often killed by passing motor vehicles.

In some areas the winter temperatures drop so markedly that snakes need to go into hibernation. A peak of activity usually precedes hibernation, during which time the snakes feed regularly in order to build up their fat reserves. Snakes may hibernate in underground burrows, under rocks or in deserted termite mounds. In very cold areas they go into full hibernation and will remain there throughout most of the winter without food or water. In other areas they may go into semi-hibernation, emerging on warm, sunny days to bask for a while but not making any attempt to feed.

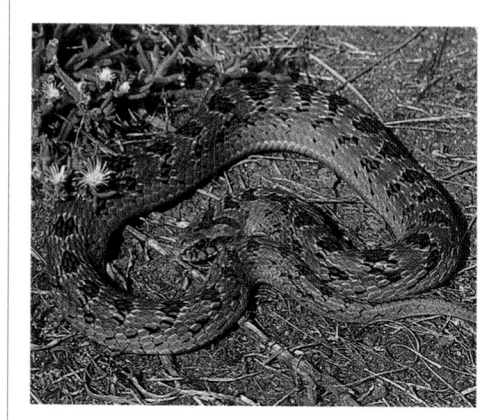

Snakes are cold-blooded and bask in the sun to raise their body temperature.

6

Individuals from different species may hibernate together. In the USA thousands of rattlesnakes hibernate together, emerging in masses once the weather heats up.

SNAKES IN THE GARDEN

Snakes are still very common in gardens, depending on where you live, how built-up the area is and how 'snake-friendly' your garden is. Some snakes, like the Brown House Snake and the Red-lipped or Herald Snake, have adapted well to urbanisation and are very at home in gardens.

Despite what you may have heard, there are no plants that keep snakes out of your garden, although certain conditions may make it more suitable for them to take up residence in an area. Piles of bricks, building rubble, compost and sheets of corrugated iron and asbestos may attract prey items such as rodents and toads, and also provide suitable hiding places for snakes. Fishponds and rockeries could add to your problems as they also attract food and provide suitable shelter for a variety of snake species. Snakes do not like large open spaces, even if they are dark. They prefer small holes or crevices where they can squeeze in tightly.

The tree-living varieties, like the bush snakes and Boomslang, obviously prefer the more vegetated areas. Again, an abundance of food will attract these species. For instance, the proliferation of the virtually transparent Tropical House Geckos along the coast has resulted in many of the harmless bush snakes taking up residence in gardens. They often live in minute crevices below the corrugated roofs of outbuildings but quickly disappear when spotted. These alert little green snakes are quite harmless.

If you have chickens or a bird aviary in your garden, prepare yourself for the odd snake that will visit in search of food. If you wish to keep your garden relatively 'snake-free', take note of the following:
- Avoid storing building rubble, bricks or sheets of corrugated tin or asbestos in your garden.
- Do not provide suitable habitat for creatures such as frogs, toads or rodents. Avoid fishponds and rockeries, chicken coops and bird aviaries.
- Keep shrubs, creepers and hedges away from the house, especially from windows that open.

WHEN A SNAKE IS SPOTTED

Should you spot a snake in the garden, keep a safe distance from it, about three metres or more, but try not to lose sight of it. Snakes disappear as quickly as they appear and if you lose sight of a snake for a few minutes, you may not find it again.

Finding help in such a situation can be problematic; you may try the fire department, local municipality, traffic department, Snake Park or the police. If you have a youngster in your area with a keen interest in snakes, he or she may be your best bet.

If you cannot get anyone to assist you, your only option may be to kill the snake. Avoid using firearms: they are are extremely dangerous and are ineffective in killing snakes; there are also restrictions to using firearms in built-up areas. A shotgun is effective but could do a great deal of damage, so if you are going to use one, do so carefully. You can kill a snake using any long object, a broomstick or a golf club, for instance: approach the snake carefully (wear eye protection – it could be a spitting snake) and give it one or two hard blows on the body. This will break the spine and kill the snake. Do not touch the seemingly dead snake as some – like the Rinkhals – play dead and the moment you get close may quickly lash out in an attempt to bite. Should you want to have the dead snake identified, carefully lift it into a bucket or cardboard box, using a stick, and take it along to the closest Snake Park or museum for positive identification.

Do bear in mind that there will only be a few common snakes in your area and it will be well worth your while getting to know these snakes.

The harmless Natal Green Snake

SNAKE BITE

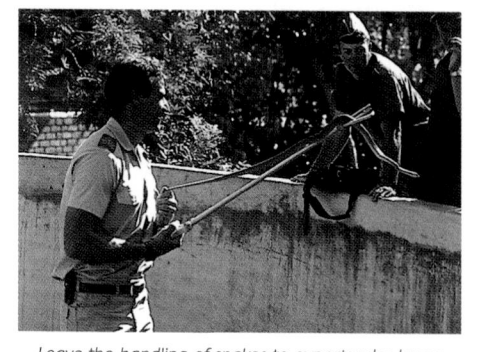

A snake bite can be serious and life threatening, and requires swift and appropriate treatment of the victim. It is certainly one instance in which 'Prevention is better than cure'. The following suggestions will help prevent the occurrence.

- Leave snakes alone and treat all snakes with respect at all times.
- Never handle small 'harmless-looking' snakes, especially those carried into your house by cats.
- Never tamper with seemingly dead snakes as many species have the nasty habit of playing dead when scared or threatened, only to strike out the moment an opportunity arises.
- Wear denim trousers and boots that cover your ankles if you spend a great deal of time outdoors. This applies to hikers, birders, fishermen and hunters. Very few snakes will successfully strike through loose-fitting denim trousers.
- Step *onto* logs and rocks, never *over* them. Snakes often sun themselves on the sides of rocks or logs.
- Never put your hand in out of reach places, especially when mountain climbing. Berg Adders often bask on small ledges and will certainly bite if a hand suddenly appears from nowhere.
- Never walk with bare feet or without a torch at night when camping or visiting a game lodge. Many snakes are active after sunset, and slow-moving species like the Puff Adder are easily trodden on.
- Do not try to kill a snake if you come across one in the wild. Throwing rocks at snakes or shooting at them is looking for trouble.

Snake-bite symptoms

Being bitten by a snake is often not immediately painful, as it usually happens very quickly. Symptoms vary dramatically from bite to bite, depending on the snake responsible for the bite and the amount of venom injected. Most venomous snakes have full control over the amount of venom they inject, and some often bite people without injecting any venom whatsoever. In snake park accidents, such bites are referred to as 'dry bites'.

Leave the handling of snakes to experts who know what they are doing.

> Surprisingly enough, many of the reported snake bites are on amateur snake handlers who have handled venomous snakes that were not correctly identified in the first place. Great care must be taken when handling all snakes and at no stage should venomous snakes be handled by people not qualified to do so.

Snake bite victims often report having seen a snake yet not knowing whether they have been bitten. The bite mark seldom resembles a 'typical' snake bite wound with two distinct fang punctures, and many consist of a single scratch or one puncture mark with a bit of bleeding.

As different snakes have different types of venom, symptoms will vary. Reactions may include:

- an immediate burning pain followed by swelling (most adders and spitting cobras).
- dizziness, difficulty in swallowing and breathing (most cobras and mambas). The latter symptoms may not appear immediately after the bite except in serious bites, especially those from the Black Mamba.
- shock, as seen in excessive sweating, a thumping heart and difficulty in breathing.

If, after several hours, symptoms include severe headaches, bleeding from small cuts and the mucous membranes and eventually severe internal bleeding, the bite may be from a Boomslang or Twig Snake.

Antivenom

The South African Institute for Medical Research in Johannesburg produces two antivenoms against the venoms of our snakes. A polyvalent antivenom (containing antibodies from more than one snake species) is produced that is effective against the venoms of most of our dangerous snakes, including the mambas, cobras and the dangerous adders but excluding the Boomslang, the Twig Snake and the Yellow-bellied Sea Snake.

The second, monovalent antivenom (containing antibodies from one strain of a single species) is effective against the venom of the Boomslang and is only available from the South African Institute of Medical Research in real emergencies.

Snake-bite outfits, containing two ampoules (20 ml) of polyvalent antivenom, can be purchased from some snake parks, pharmacies and from the South African Institute of Medical Research. This must be stored in a refrigerator (but should not be frozen) as it will lose its clarity and potency if exposed to high temperatures for extended periods of time. If you have any intention of administering antivenom in an emergency, discuss the use thereof with a doctor or authority on the treatment of snake bite.

Antivenom is most effective if injected intravenously and in fairly large quantities (40–60 ml). This is potentially dangerous, as some people (especially those with a history of allergies) are sensitive to antivenom. Ideally, someone who has experience and the necessary drugs to combat adverse reactions (which may develop rapidly) should administer it. Intramuscular or subcutaneous administration of antivenom is far less effective than the intravenous route but may delay serious symptoms until the victim reaches proper medical help. Antivenom should not be injected near the site of the bite.

Generally, you should avoid injecting antivenom except in known cases of bites by the Black or Green mambas, the Cape Cobra, Snouted Cobra, Forest Cobra and the Mozambique Spitting Cobra (*not* for the Rinkhals). Early intravenous administration of antivenom in such cases might save the victim's life. Always study the pamphlet in any snake-bite kit before injecting antivenom.

FIRST-AID

Cutting of the area surrounding a snake-bite wound and sucking out venom, as seen in many a Wild West movie, is certainly not a recommended first-aid measure. Similarly, the use of a tourniquet that cuts off blood circulation is no longer recommended as it may cause unnecessary pain and even tissue damage (known in the past to result in the loss of limbs). There is also no evidence to suggest that the application of electrical current (sometimes applied with a cattle prodder) neutralises the effects of snake venom. Bear in mind that the snake responsible for the bite may even have been harmless!

The best first-aid measure in the event of a snake bite is the use of pressure or 'crepe' bandages, which are very effective and have no detrimental effects.

First-aid procedures

Remove the victim's shoes but do not waste time removing clothing.

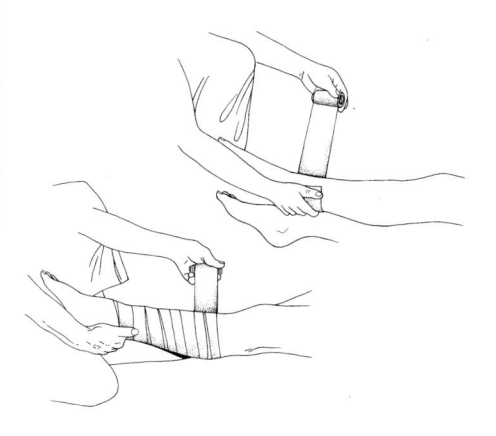

Apply firm pressure to the site of the bite, using your hand. Then wrap the limb firmly with a crepe bandage (tear up some clothing if a bandage is not available), starting at the site of the bite and working towards the heart.

You are not trying to cut off blood circulation but rather to prevent venom being absorbed through the lymphatic system. The bandage must be quite tight, as for a sprained ankle.

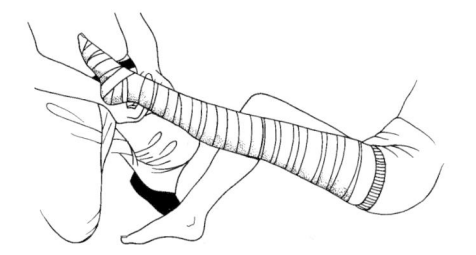

Apply the bandage over the entire limb if possible.

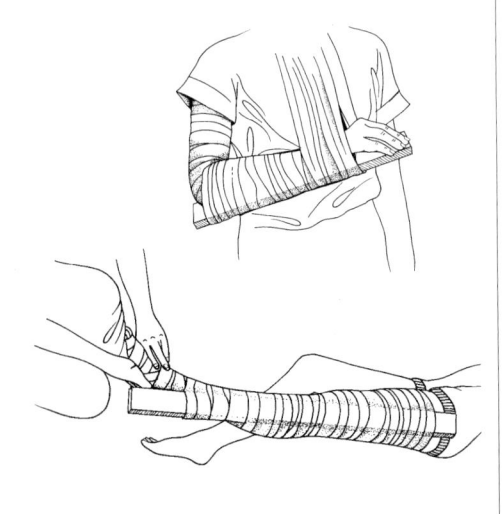

Immobilise the victim and, if possible, splint the limb. If there is severe swelling, the bandage must be loosened but *not* removed.

Lay the victim down (unnecessary movement increases venom circulation) and keep him/her calm and reassured.

Transport the victim to the closest hospital. If there is no hospital closeby, transport the victim to the closest doctor.

Also important to note:
- Do not inject antivenom indiscriminately. This should be left for a doctor.
- Do not give the victim alcohol or any other liquid.
- Keep the mouth and throat clear of saliva and resort to artificial respiration if necessary.

- Suction may help if done immediately, even if only to reassure the victim. All fluid removed by suction must be spat out immediately. If possible, suck over a sheet of rubber or plastic.
- Do not try to kill the snake responsible. A second bite would really complicate matters.
- Keep your wits about you and react in a logical way. Remember that very few people die from snake bite.

A snake bite victim should be hospitalised for at least two days. In the event of a serious bite, antivenom is very effective and should be administered. It is usually used in conjunction with intravenous cortisone and sometimes with adrenaline. It is best to leave such specialised treatment to the medical profession, if you have the choice.

SPITTING SNAKES

Snakes spit (or rather 'squirt') their venom in self-defence, to keep predators at bay, or to scare off humans that venture too close. This is done by applying pressure on the venom glands, so forcing the venom down the hollow fangs. A small hole near the tip of the fangs forces the venom out of the snake's mouth. A spitting snake can eject its venom as far as 2,5 metres and sometimes even further. This spitting action is not very accurate (snake's do not 'aim') but it is effective.

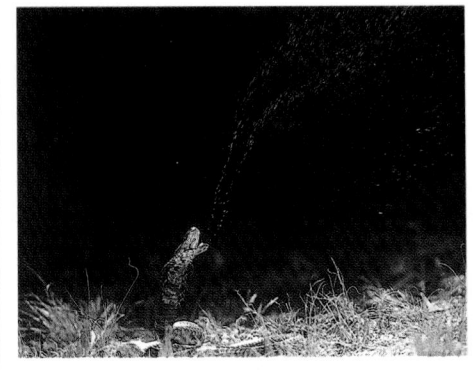

A Mozambique Spitting Cobra ejects its venom.

There are two common spitting snakes in southern Africa, the Rinkhals and the Mozambique Spitting Cobra. Two other lesser-known and less common 'spitters' are the Black Spitting Cobra and the Western Barred Spitting Cobra.

Snake venom is completely harmless to the skin unless it enters an open wound. In the eyes, however, it is absorbed rapidly by tiny blood vessels close to the surface and causes severe burning and inflammation. Rubbing the eyes does further harm.

First-aid procedures for venom in the eyes

■ Rinse the eyes immediately with large quantities of water or any other harmless fluid such as milk, or even beer.

■ Wipe any excess venom from the face.

■ Seek medical advice. It may be necessary for a doctor to rinse the eyes with diluted antivenom (one part serum to nine parts water).

The victim's eyes should recover fully within three or four days.

HABITATS OF SOUTHERN AFRICA

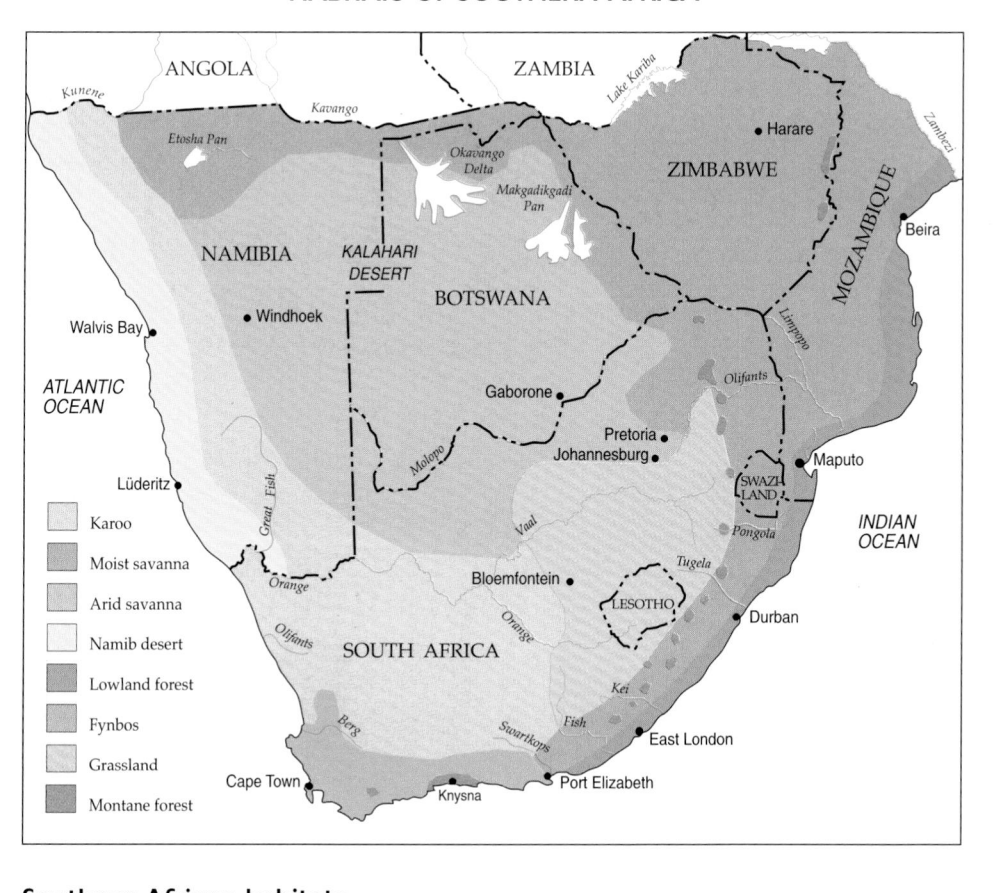

Southern African habitats

A habitat is the particular environment in which an organism lives. Southern Africa has eight distinct habitats or vegetation types in which snakes (and other wildlife) may be found. These are depicted on the map above.

HOW TO USE THIS BOOK

This guide to the snakes of southern Africa is intended as a practical tool to the easy identification of all the region's dangerous and common harmless snakes. Its other important purpose is to provide quick and practical advice on first-aid measures, should someone get bitten.

Within the accounts that follow, each species is introduced by its English common name, followed by its scientific name and an indication as to whether the snake is harmless, mildly venomous, dangerous or very dangerous. Alternative English common names and the Afrikaans name(s), appear at the top of the left-hand column, and simple icons convey additional information about the snake:

■ average size – shown relative to an average human male of I, 8 metres tall, or to an average human arm of 60 cm.

  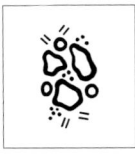

60 cm	1,8 metres

■ whether the snake lives mostly in trees, in shrubs, on the ground, or any combination of the three.

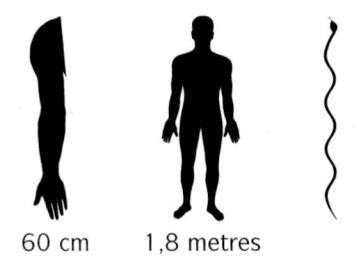

tree-dwelling	shrub-dwelling	ground-dwelling

■ whether the snake is active during the day (diurnal), at night (nocturnal), or both.

nocturnal	diurnal

A separate '**Look out for**' column highlights each snake's most prominent features, be that body markings, diagnostic signs or behaviour. This assists in easily identifying a specific snake species.

Colour photographs have been used unsparingly, especially where several colour forms exist or where snakes differ in colour according to region. Photographs of similar or easily confused species are also featured along with the snake under discussion to rule out confusion between species.

While every effort has been made to avoid technical language, some technical terms have been necessary; these are explained in the Glossary, which appears on page 86.

The 42 snakes featured in this book have been grouped according to four snake types: the adders (pages 14-25); the elapids (pages 26-47), the back-fanged snakes (page 48-67), and the fangless and non-poisonous snakes (pages 68-85).

ADDERS are very common throughout the region and are found in or close to most major cities. They also account for many of the serious snake-bite cases that

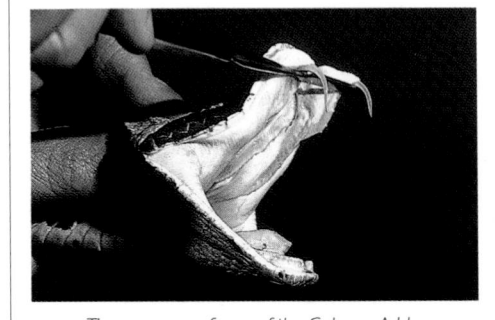

The enormous fangs of the Gaboon Adder.

are reported (the Puff Adder at the top of the list). With the exception of the Night Adder, most adders are short and fat with the head distinct from the rest of the body.

Adders have large fangs situated in the front of the mouth. When the fangs are not in use they fold back against the roof of the mouth. Most have cytotoxic or cell-destroying venoms that are responsible for the destruction of tissue and blood vessels. Symptoms are localised and bites are often very painful, followed by severe swelling and occasionally blistering. Fortunately, bites from small adders are not usually too serious, although they may be very painful. Most adders (except the Night Adder) are viviparous or live-bearing.

ELAPIDS are venomous snakes with fixed grooved fangs in the front of the mouth; they include the cobras and mambas and related snakes. Of all southern African elapids, the cobras, mambas, Rinkhals and the sea snake possess the most potent venoms. All of the remaining elapids are venomous, though most not dangerously so.

Most elapids are long and slender. The Rinkhals and the cobras are easily identified as they rear their heads off the ground and spread a hood. The two mambas are both rather elusive and infrequently seen.

The venom of most cobras, the Rinkhals and the mambas is primarily neurotoxic, affecting the nervous system. The onset of symptoms is rapid and may include dizziness, difficulty in swallowing, slurred speech, blurred vision and eventually unconsciousness. In untreated cases, death follows after about eight hours or more, usually as a result of respiratory failure. Most elapids are oviparous or egg-laying, excepting the Rinkhals – which is viviparous.

BACK-FANGED SNAKES are snakes with small fangs on the upper jaw, more or less behind the eye. Of all the back-fanged snakes only the Boomslang and Twig Snake are known to have very potent venoms that are of medical significance. They possess haemotoxic venoms which affect the blood-clotting mechanism, causing severe headaches, bleeding from the mucous membranes, nausea, vomiting and eventually bleeding from all internal organs. The onset of symptoms may be slow – anything from 8-24 hours or even longer.

The majority of back-fanged snakes are long and slender, and are oviparous or egg-laying.

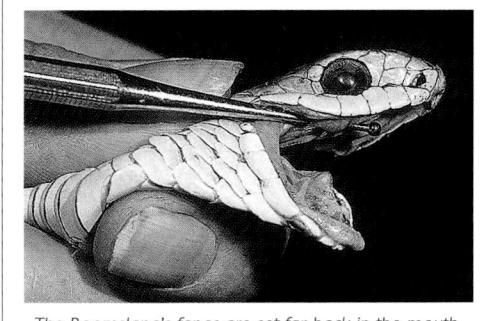

The Boomslang's fangs are set far back in the mouth.

FANGLESS AND NON-POISONOUS SNAKES do not possess venom, but they do have teeth and some of them, particularly the African Rock Python and large Mole Snakes, are capable of inflicting painful bites.

Most of the fangless snakes are oviparous or egg-laying, the Mole Snake and slug-eaters being exceptions.

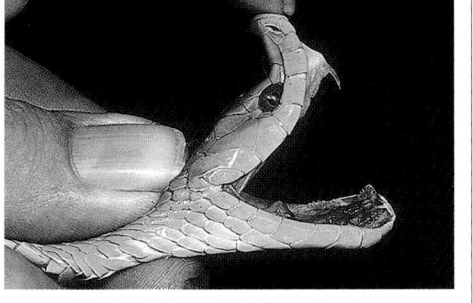

The short fangs of the Green Mamba.

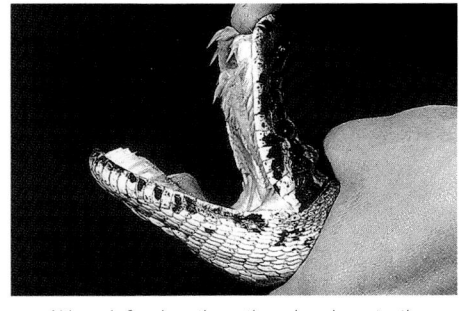

Although fangless, the python does have teeth.

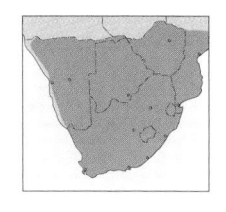

PUFF ADDER
Bitis arietans

Other names
Pofadder (A)

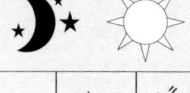

Average 90 cm
Maximum 1,7 m

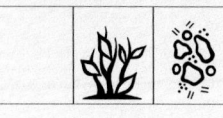

LOOK OUT FOR
- A short, stubby snake with a triangular head distinct from the rest of the body.
- Yellow to grey-brown with distinct black chevrons on the back.
- May hiss or puff when disturbed.
- Usually found on the ground.
- Very active after sunset.

Preferred habitat
Common throughout most of southern Africa except for mountain tops, true desert and dense forests. It does not occur in and around the Johannesburg region.

Habits
A slow-moving, bad-tempered and excitable snake that may hiss or puff when disturbed. Usually found on the ground but it may venture onto small shrubs to sun itself. Mainly active at night, often basking on tarred roads, where it may be killed by passing vehicles.

It relies on its perfect camouflage to escape detection and will rather freeze than move off. People often step onto or close to Puff Adders and then get bitten. Like most other snakes, this snake swims well.

Similar species
May be confused with the Gaboon Adder or some of the smaller adders. Note: None of the harmless snakes resemble the Puff Adder.

Enemies
Man, warthogs, birds of prey and other snakes (e.g. Snouted Cobra).

Food and feeding
Usually ambushes its prey. It feeds on rats and mice, other small terrestrial

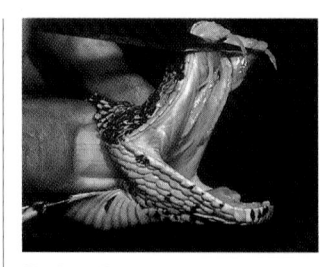

The long fangs inject a potent venom.

mammals, ground birds, lizards, toads and occasionally other snakes. Rodents are usually bitten and left to die. The Puff Adder then follows its prey's scent with a flickering tongue. The prey is swallowed head first.

Reproduction
Viviparous, giving birth in late summer to 20-40 young, though exceptional broods of 80 have been recorded. The young, measuring 15-20 cm, are born in a fine membranous sac from which they break free soon after birth. Large individuals from East Africa are known to produce more than 150 young, the largest number of any snake species in the world.

People are at risk of stepping onto Puff Adders at night as they often move about slowly once the sun has set.

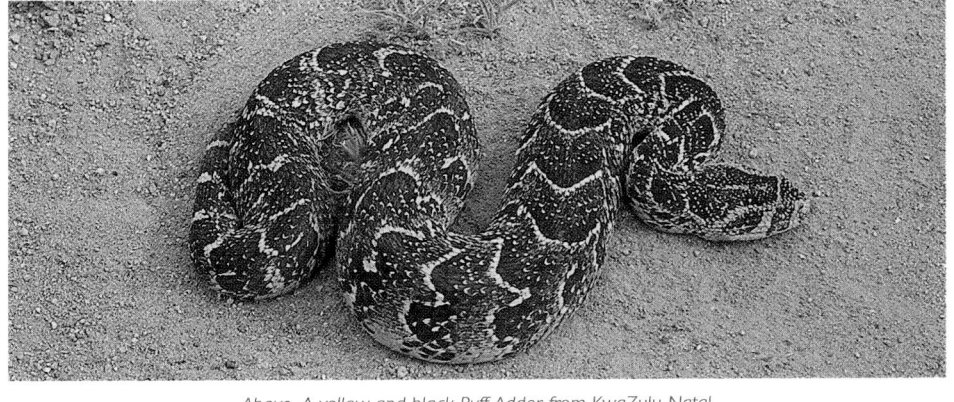

Above: A yellow and black Puff Adder, from KwaZulu-Natal.
Opposite, centre: A dull-coloured Puff Adder from the Northern Province.

Danger to man

Because of its reliance on camouflage to escape detection, this bad-tempered snake with its long fangs (up to 18 mm) and potent venom features prominently in snake-bite accidents. The Puff Adder accounts for about 60 % of serious snake bites in southern Africa. Although few of these bites prove fatal, this snake is still responsible for the majority of snake-bite deaths in this region.

Venom

A potent cytotoxic or cell-destroying venom that attacks tissue and blood cells. Other than immediate shock, symptoms include extreme pain, excessive swelling and sometimes blistering at the site of the bite. Most victims are bitten on the lower leg. Fortunately, the venom is slow-acting, taking up to 24 hours or even more to cause death if not treated or if treatment is unsuccessful. It is uncommon for victims to die in a shorter period of time. With fatal bites, the victims usually succumb to complications associated with extensive swelling or kidney failure. Antivenom will be required in serious cases.

First-aid procedures

- Immobilise and reassure the patient, who must lie down and be kept as quiet as possible.
- Apply a pressure bandage immediately (*see* page 9) and immobilise the limb with a splint to reduce the spread of venom.
- Loosen, but do not remove, the bandage if there is severe swelling.
- Transport promptly to hospital.

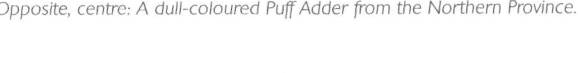

A dull-coloured Puff Adder, from Namibia.

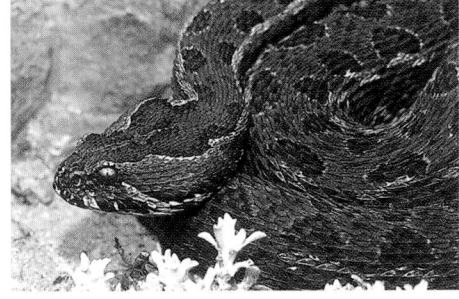

The Berg Adder is differently patterned to the Puff Adder.

15

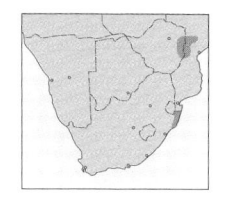

GABOON ADDER

Bitis gabonica

Other names
Gaboenadder (A)

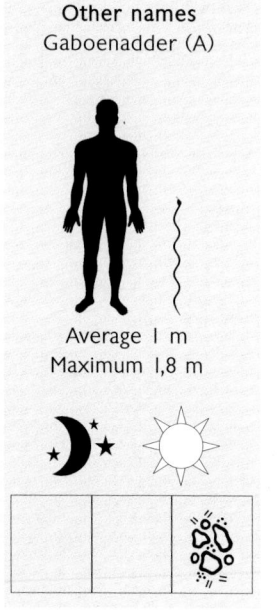

Average 1 m
Maximum 1,8 m

LOOK OUT FOR
- A fat snake with a triangular head which is very distinct from the rest of the body.
- Beautiful colours in various shades of dark and light brown, buff, purple and pink.
- Huffs and puffs a great deal when disturbed.
- Always found on the ground.
- Mainly active at night.

Preferred habitat
In southern Africa it prefers moist, thickly wooded lowland areas in coastal dune and forests on the eastern escarpment of Zimbabwe. The Gaboon Adder has a restricted distribution within its range.

Habits
Though mainly active at night it may be seen basking in the sun on a forest floor. It is a sluggish snake that may remain in one spot for days. Compared with the Puff Adder it is surprisingly placid in nature. When disturbed it will emit a series of long, drawn-out hisses while the forepart of the body is lifted off the ground horizontally. Even then it is reluctant to strike.

Similar species
May be confused with the Puff Adder but is far more colourful and more impressively patterned.

Enemies
Much of this snake's habitat in northern Zululand has been destroyed by squatters. Many individuals are also captured by snake enthusiasts, usually while crossing roads at night. The Gaboon Adder is rare in northern Zululand and is listed as vulnerable in the latest *South African Red Data Book - Reptiles and Amphibians.*

Food and feeding
May hunt from dusk onwards, otherwise ambushes its prey. Unlike the Puff Adder, it tends to hang onto its prey while the venom takes effect. Favourite prey includes rodents, hares, ground birds and toads. Small monkeys and duiker are also taken.

Reproduction
Viviparous, giving birth to 16-30 young (in South Africa) in late summer, measuring 25-32 cm in length. The young are perfect replicas of the adults.

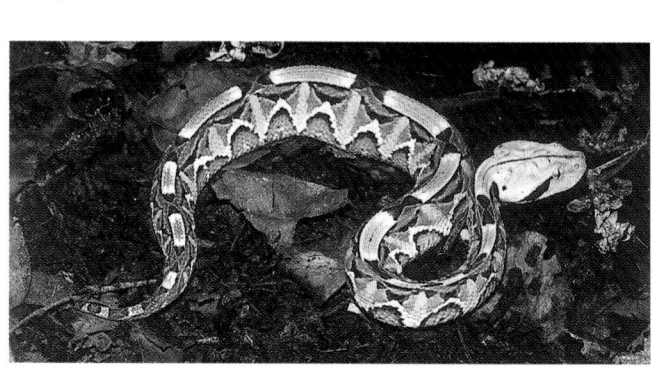

The Gaboon Adder is far more colourfully marked than the Puff Adder.

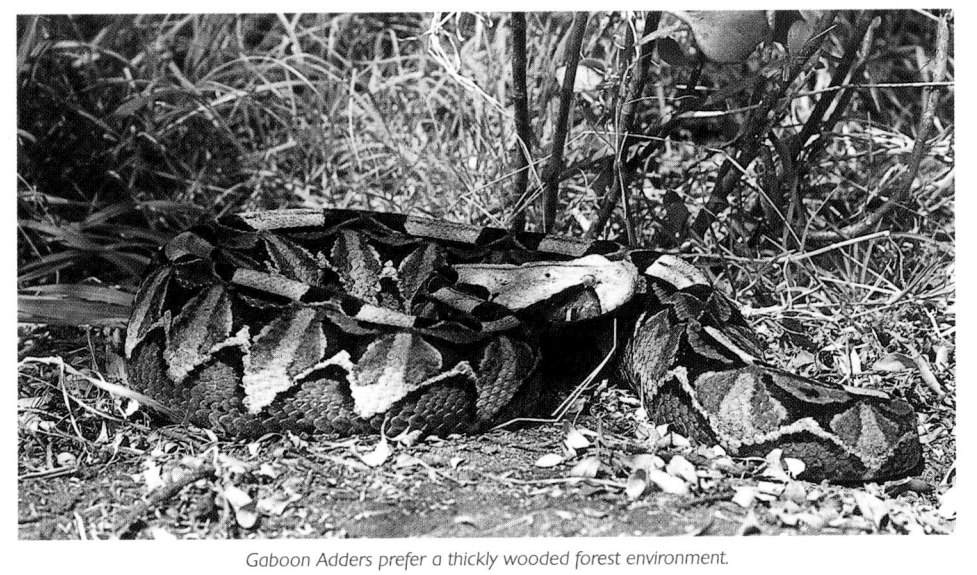

Gaboon Adders prefer a thickly wooded forest environment.

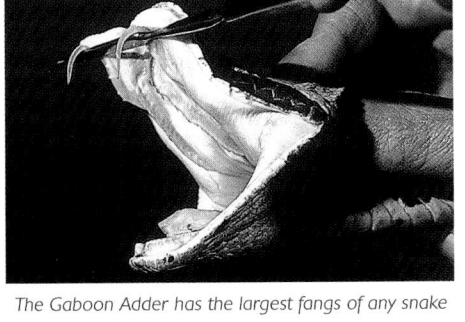

The Gaboon Adder has the largest fangs of any snake in the world.

Males are known to engage in combat during autumn and early winter. This snake is known to hybridise with the Puff Adder. A single hybrid, measuring 1,24 m, was found near Mtubatuba in 1972.

This snake, despite its complex coloration, is perfectly camouflaged among leaf litter and can easily be trodden on. It is rare throughout most of its range, and bites are seldom reported.

Danger to man

This snake has a potent cytotoxic venom and can inject large quantities in a single bite. It also has enormous fangs that grow up to 40 mm in length. It is extremely dangerous to man but is rarely encountered. Very few bites are reported.

Venom

The potently cytotoxic venom is comparable with that of the Puff Adder, but much larger quantities may be injected in a single bite. A full bite from a Gaboon Adder will result in alarming symptoms and early death unless treated promptly with antivenom. The victim must be treated for shock immediately. Symptoms may include severe pain, swelling and necrosis.

First-aid procedures

- Immobilise and reassure the patient, who must lie down and be kept as quiet as possible.
- Apply a pressure bandage immediately (*see* page 9) and immobilise the limb with a splint to reduce the spread of venom.
- Loosen, but do not remove, the bandage if there is severe swelling.
- Transport promptly to hospital.

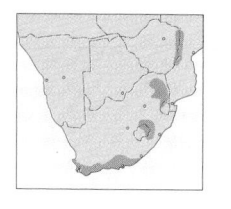

BERG ADDER

Bitis atropos

Other names
Bergadder (A)

Average 30 cm
Maximum 60 cm

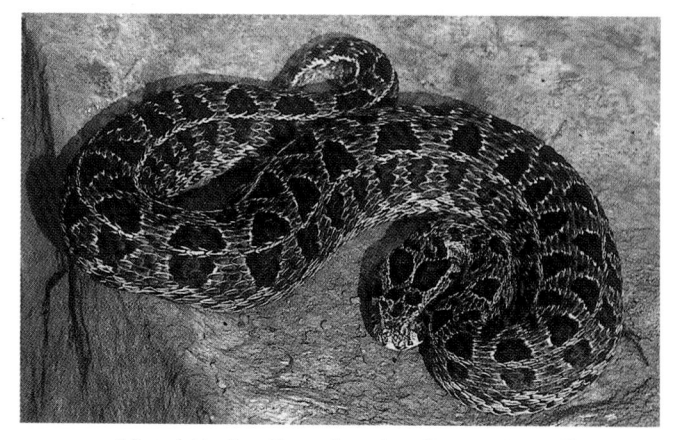

A Berg Adder from the south-western Cape sunning itself.

LOOK OUT FOR
- A triangular head distinct from the rest of the body.
- Lacks chevron markings along the body as seen in the Puff Adder (*see* p.14).
- Hisses loudly when encountered.
- Strikes readily, even when the aggressor is well out of reach.
- Likes to bask in the sun.

Preferred habitat

Montane grassland, fynbos and rocky slopes from sea level in the Eastern, Western and Northern Cape, up to 3 000 m in the Drakensberg.

Habits

A particularly bad-tempered snake that hisses loudly and will strike readily if approached. It is frequently found basking in grass tussocks, on rocky ledges or on footpaths and will quickly seek refuge if disturbed.

Similar species

May be confused with the Puff Adder. Its triangular head is distinct from the body and, like the Puff Adder, it hisses when encountered.

Enemies

Predatory birds and other snakes.

Food and feeding

Mainly lizards and small rodents but also amphibians, including rain frogs. Nestlings of ground-living birds and smaller snakes are also taken. Juveniles, however, feed largely on frogs and other amphibians.

Reproduction

Mating occurs in autumn and the females give birth to 4-15 young in late summer. The young measure from 9-15 cm in length. Females are known to produce more than one batch of young from a single mating.

Danger to man

Berg Adders are common, like to bask in the sun and strike readily when encountered. Bites may result in minor neurological symptoms but no fatalities are known.

18

Venom

The venom differs from that of most adders in that it is mildly neurotoxic, with a specific action on the optic and facial nerves, causing drooping eyelids, dizziness and temporary loss of taste and smell. Unlike cobra venom, it is not known to cause difficulty in breathing. Most victims recover fully within a few days. Patients should be treated symptomatically. Few bites result in swelling and necrosis. Antivenom does not neutralise the venom of this snake and therefore is not required. Though no deaths have been recorded, bites may be serious and should be treated as such.

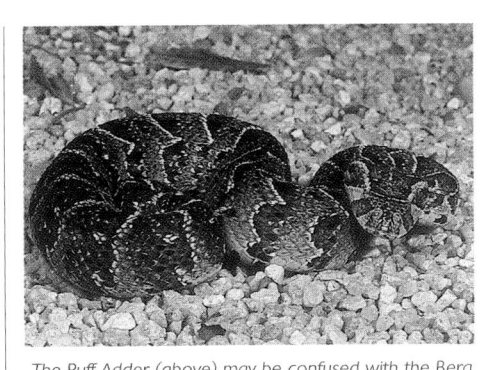

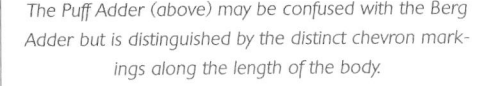

The Puff Adder (above) may be confused with the Berg Adder but is distinguished by the distinct chevron markings along the length of the body.

Mountaineers and hikers are at risk, particularly when reaching up to ledges which are out of sight. Boots provide adequate protection against the bite of this snake.

First-aid procedures

- Immobilise and reassure the patient, who must lie down and be kept as quiet as possible.
- Apply a pressure bandage immediately (*see page 9*) and immobilise the limb with a splint to reduce the spread of venom.
- Loosen, but do not remove, the bandage if there is severe swelling.
- Transport promptly to hospital.

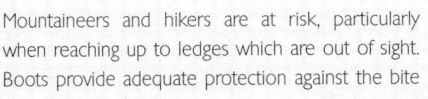

A dull-coloured Berg Adder.

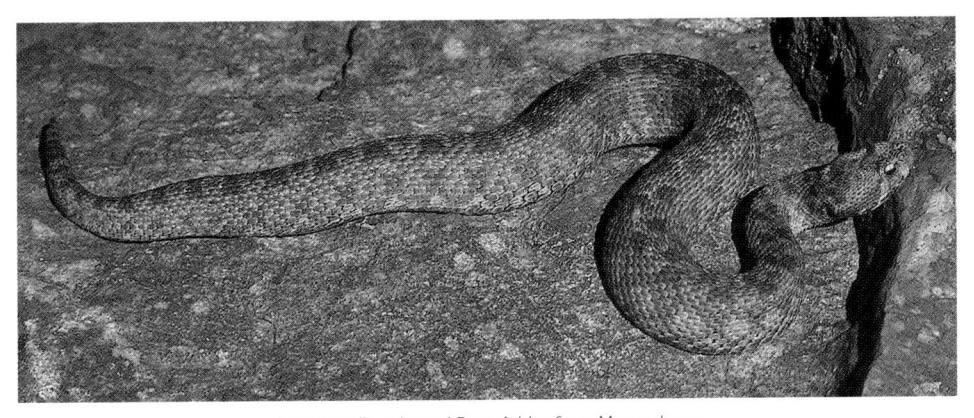

An unusually coloured Berg Adder from Mpumalanga.

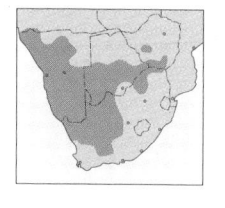

HORNED ADDER

Bitis caudalis

Other names
Horingadder;
Horingsman (A)

Average 25 cm
Maximum 50 cm

LOOK OUT FOR
- A small adder with a triangular head distinct from the rest of the body.
- A single horn above each eye.
- Hisses and strikes readily.
- May worm itself into loose sand with only parts of the head exposed.

Preferred habitat
Dry, sandy regions in the Namib Desert, Karoo and arid savanna.

Habits
A small adder that may bury itself in loose sand by wriggling or shuffling until concealed. Only the top of the head, the eyes and the little horns are left exposed. Like Peringuey's Adder, this snake may also sidewind on loose sand.

When disturbed, it may coil, inflate its body with air and hiss loudly, often striking repeatedly. The Horned Adder is most active at dusk, prior to which it prefers to lie in the shade of shrubs or rocks.

Similar species
The Horned Adder may resemble a small Puff Adder but can be distinguished by its small horns, one above

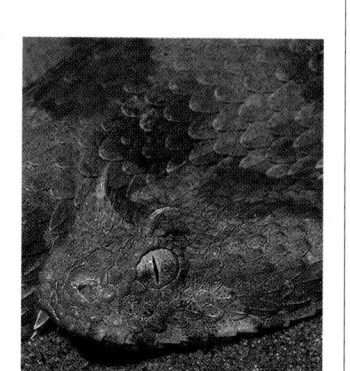

A reddish-coloured Horned Adder from Sesriem in Namibia.

each eye. May also be confused with other small adders like the Many-horned Adder or the Plain Mountain Adder as well as the harmless Dwarf Beaked Snake.

Enemies
Predatory birds and other snakes. Also humans as it is very popular in private collections.

Food and feeding
Feeds on small lizards such as skinks, which it ambushes in the day, or geckos and small rodents, which it hunts at night. Amphibians are also taken. The Horned Adder uses the darkened tip of its tail to lure lizards closer when it is buried in loose sand. When it strikes, it hangs onto its prey while its venom takes effect.

This snake is most active at dusk. It hisses and strikes readily and may be heard hissing long before it is seen. Boots provide adequate protection against its bite.

Reproduction
Viviparous, giving birth to 4-8 or as many as 19 young which are born during summer or early autumn, more or less at the same time that many lizards' eggs hatch. The newborn young measure from 11-15 cm in length.

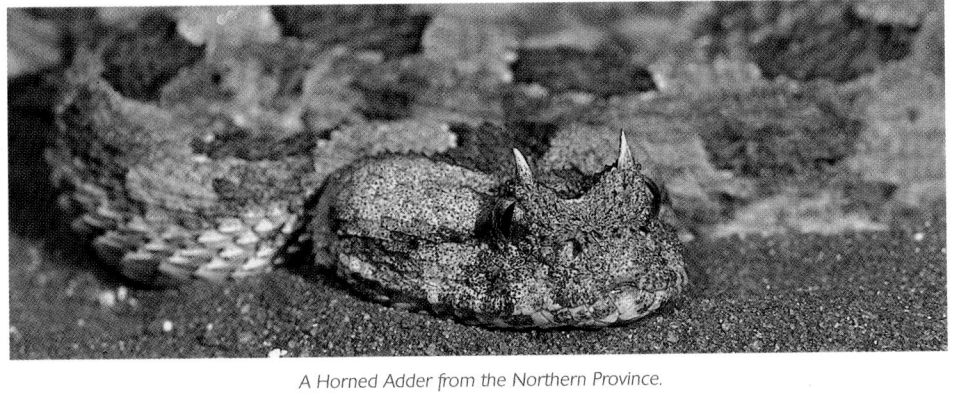
A Horned Adder from the Northern Province.

Danger to man

May inflict a painful bite which causes swelling and some necrosis, but poses no real threat to man.

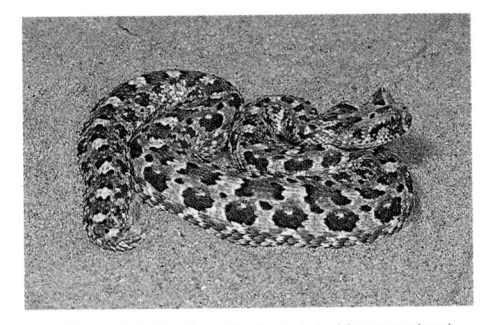
A Horned Adder from Springbok in Namaqualand.

Venom

The venom is mildly cytotoxic causing swelling and much pain, accompanied by shock and local necrosis. It is not known to be fatal and antivenom is not required. Healing may take several weeks.

First-aid procedures

If you are absolutely sure that the Horned Adder was responsible for the bite:

- Get the victim to a doctor or hospital where the bite must be treated symptomatically.
- Otherwise resort to first-aid measures (page 9).

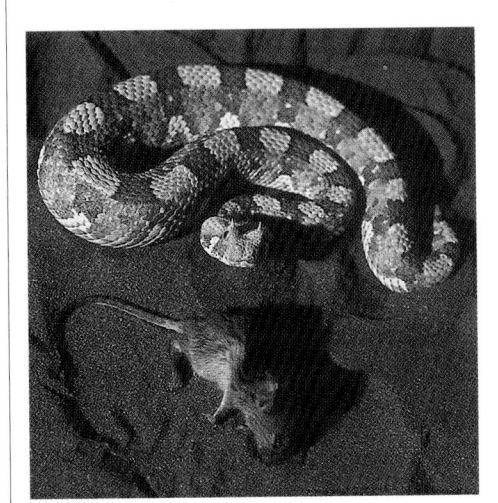

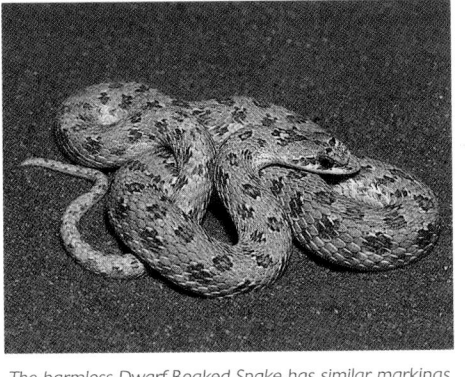
The harmless Dwarf Beaked Snake has similar markings.

A Horned Adder with prey.

MANY-HORNED ADDER

Bitis cornuta

DANGEROUS

Other names
Veelhoringadder;
Horingsman (A)

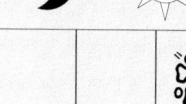

Average 30 cm
Maximum 61 cm

Preferred habitat
Found on mountains, rocky outcrops and gravel plains in the Namib Desert and in arid savanna.

Habits
Though this snake is capable of sidewinding and burying itself in loose sand, it prefers rocky areas on sandy or gravel flats where it can easily shelter from the wind. It is most active at dusk or in the early mornings. When confronted, it will hiss loudly and strike with so much force that most of its body will lift off the ground.

Similar species
May be confused with a young Puff Adder or some of the smaller adders such as the Horned Adder, but is distinguished by the tuft of 2-4 horns on either side of the head, above each eye.

Enemies
Preyed upon by other snakes. Many individuals are captured for the exotic pet trade and exported illegally. Also, often killed by passing vehicles when crossing roads.

> The Many-horned Adder will hiss loudly and strike viciously when confronted. Boots provide adequate protection against the bite of this snake.

LOOK OUT FOR
- A tuft of 2-4 horns above each eye.
- Often seen crossing roads after sunset.
- Prefers gravel flats where it can shelter from the wind.
- Most active at dusk and in the early mornings.

A Many-horned Adder from Lüderitz, Namibia.

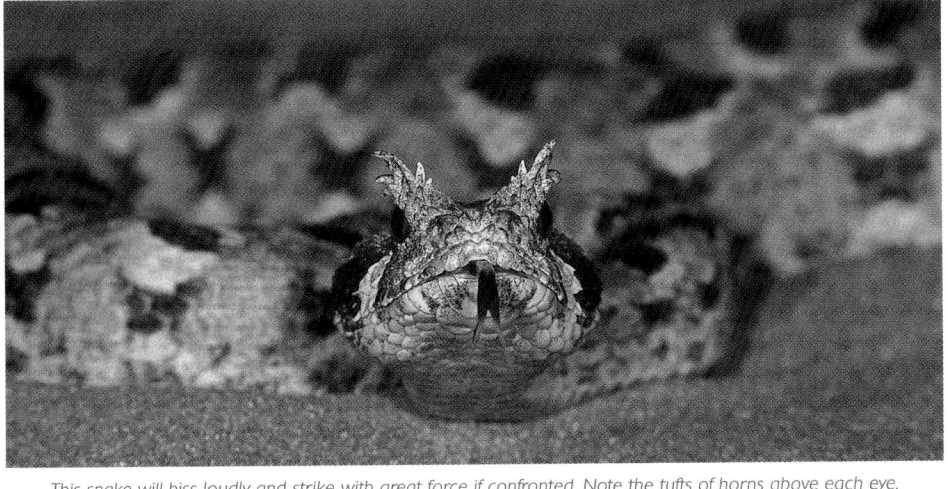

This snake will hiss loudly and strike with great force if confronted. Note the tufts of horns above each eye.

Food and feeding

Feeds mainly on ground-living lizards, small rodents and amphibians.

Reproduction

Viviparous, giving birth to 7-12 young in late summer or early autumn. The young measure 13-15 cm in length.

Did you know?

Snakes do not need to feed regularly and can survive several months without eating. Warm-blooded creatures, such as mammals and birds, need regular meals to maintain a constant body temperature. Reptiles, on the other hand, rely on their immediate environment for their heat requirements. In winter, snakes may go into hibernation and will refrain from eating for up to six or seven months with no ill effects.

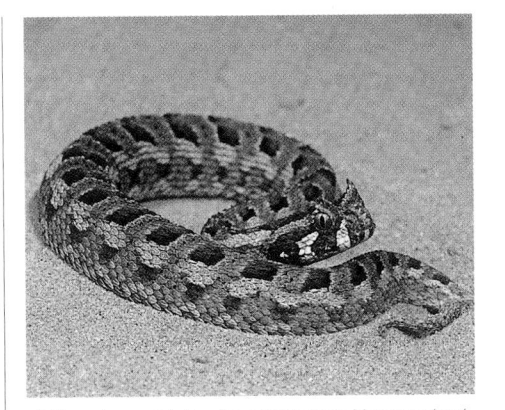

A Many-horned Adder from Springbok, Namaqualand.

Venom

Mildly cytotoxic with much pain and swelling accompanied by necrosis. It is not known to be fatal and anti-venom is not required.

First-aid procedures

If you are sure of the identity of the snake:

- Get the victim to a doctor or hospital where the bite must be treated symptomatically.
- Painkillers will be required.
- Otherwise resort to first-aid measures (page 9).

Danger to man

The venom is supposedly as potent as that of the Puff Adder, but this snake's venom yield is minute. It poses no real threat to man, even though it is capable of inflicting an extremely painful bite.

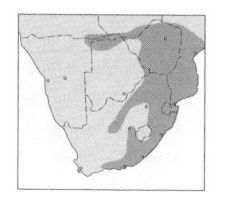

COMMON NIGHT ADDER

Causus rhombeatus

Other names
Gewone Nagadder (A)

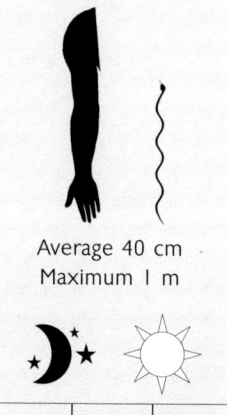

Average 40 cm
Maximum 1 m

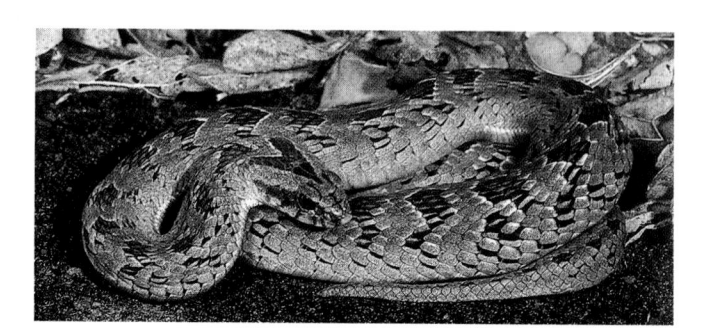

The V-shaped marking on the head, so characteristic of the Common Night Adder, is clearly visible on this specimen.

LOOK OUT FOR
- A distinct V-shaped marking on the head.
- Prefers damp areas, often close to some form of water.
- Coils up and hisses when confronted.

Preferred habitat
Favours damp environments in moist savanna, lowland forest and fynbos where it seeks refuge in old termite mounds, under logs and large flat stones, and amongst building rubble. Often found close to dams and rivers.

Did you know?
An encounter with one snake does not mean that another is lurking. Snakes are loners and as a rule move about on their own. The only time that snakes might be seen in pairs is during the mating season. However, some areas offer ideal conditions for snakes, and may provide ample hiding place and a good source of food. Under such circumstances, a number of snakes may be found within a restricted area.

Habits
A docile snake that moves off if given the choice. If cornered or provoked it will inflate its body with air, coil its body and hiss aggressively, striking violently at the same time. It is fond of basking during the day and hunts in the evenings. In its search for food the Common Night Adder will often venture close to or even into farmsteads and houses. It has very long venom glands that extend back into the neck region.

Similar species
May be confused with the harmless Rhombic Egg-eating Snake as both have similar markings. The Night Adder, however, has a short, thicker body with a flat head on which a black V-shaped marking is clearly visible. The Rhombic Egg-eater may have two or three fragmented V-shaped markings on the neck *behind* the head.

24

Enemies

Preyed upon by a number of other snakes, leguaans (or monitor lizards), and predatory birds.

Food and feeding

This snake has poor eyesight and relies heavily on smell to locate its prey. It feeds almost exclusively on toads and frogs, including the rain frog. Frequents houses to feed on toads that prey on insects attracted by light. The hatchlings are known to feed on tadpoles.

Reproduction

Oviparous, laying 12-26 eggs two or three times a year. The eggs, measuring 26-30 x 14-19 mm, stick together and form a small bundle. The young measure 13-16 cm in length. This is the only egg-laying member of the adder group.

Danger to man

The venom is only mildly cytotoxic and generally not dangerous to man. No human deaths have been recorded to date.

Venom

Cytotoxic, causing pain and swelling. May cause acute discomfort in some cases. Though antivenom is effective against the venom of this snake, it is generally not required. However, the bite of the Common Night Adder should not be treated lightly.

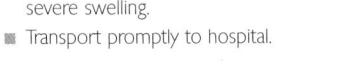

This snake hunts for food in the evenings, so take care not to accidentally stand on one.

First-aid procedures

- Immobilise and reassure the patient, who must lie down and be kept as quiet as possible.
- Apply a pressure bandage immediately (*see* page 9) and immobilise the limb with a splint to reduce the spread of venom.
- Loosen, but do not remove, the bandage if there is severe swelling.
- Transport promptly to hospital.

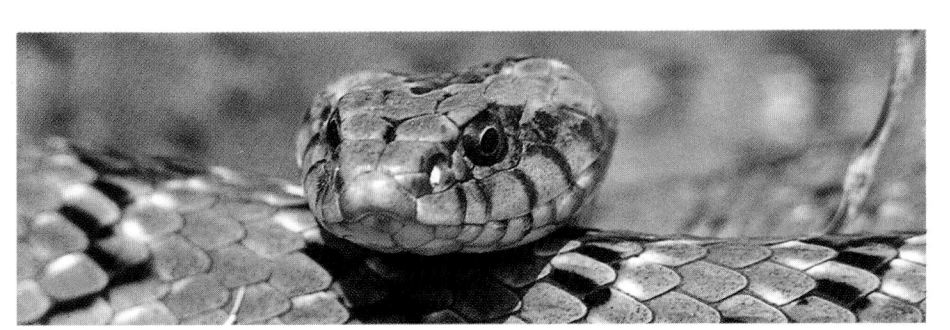

The Common Night Adder is fond of basking by day and is more active in the evening.

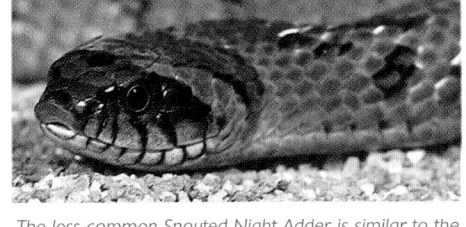

The similar-looking Rhombic Egg-eater has V-markings on the neck, not on the head.

The less common Snouted Night Adder is similar to the Common Night Adder, and is equally venomous.

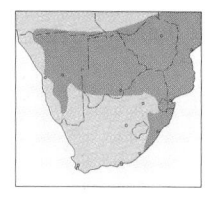

BLACK MAMBA

Dendroaspis polylepis

Other names
Swartmamba (A)

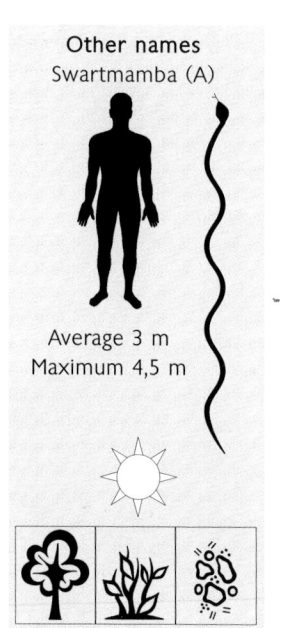

Average 3 m
Maximum 4,5 m

Preferred habitat
Termite mounds, hollow tree trunks and granite hillocks in both dry and moist savanna, and in lowland forest.

Habits
A graceful, alert and unpredictable snake with a deadly poison. It is southern Africa's largest poisonous snake. The Black Mamba is active during the day when it hunts for food. Hunting is usually done from a permanent lair to which it will return regularly if not disturbed. It is also very fond of basking and will return to the same site daily. If it senses danger, it is quick to slither away into dense undergrowth or to disappear down the nearest hole.

Equally at home in trees and on the ground, it seems to favour the ground. It is a large snake and can move comfortably with as much as one third of its body off the ground.

> This is one of the deadliest snakes in the world and should be avoided at all costs. If you come across one and retreat slowly and carefully, the snake will do the same.

The Black Mamba seldom permits a close approach (within 40 metres). If cornered or threatened it will gape, exposing the black inner lining of its mouth, and will spread a narrow

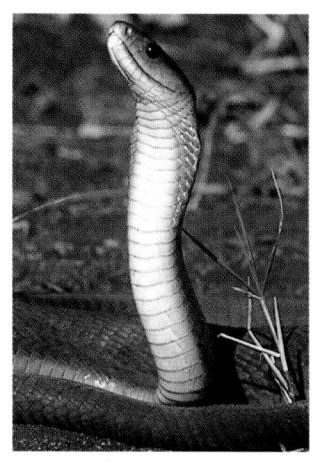

If threatened it spreads a narrow hood to make itself look bigger.

hood while waving the tongue slowly up and down. Any sudden movement at this stage will be met with a series of rapid strikes, often with fatal results.

Similar species
People tend to mistake any grey, brown or black snake for the Black Mamba. It may be confused with the larger cobras, female Boomslang, Mole Snake, Olive House Snake and some of the grass or sand snakes.

Enemies
Birds of prey and other snakes. Juvenile Black Mambas are extremely nervous and are seldom seen. They grow rapidly and can reach a length of two metres within a year. Adults have very few enemies.

LOOK OUT FOR
- Usually an overall olive-brown to grey.
- Very nervous and quick to spread a narrow hood when threatened.
- A coffin-shaped head.
- Can move with up to a third of its body well off the ground.
- Regularly basks in the same spot.
- Active during the day.

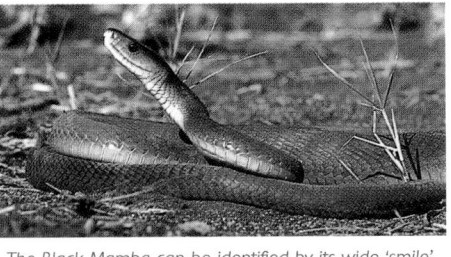

The Black Mamba can be identified by its wide 'smile'.

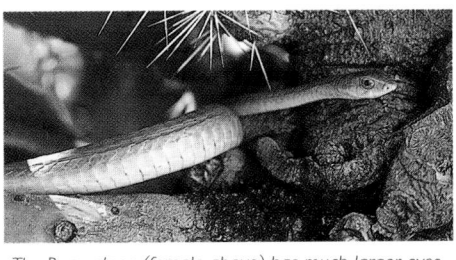

The Boomslang (female above) has much larger eyes.

Food and feeding

Actively hunts rodents, squirrels, dassies and other suitably sized mammals, as well as fledgling birds. The prey is bitten once or twice and quickly succumbs to the potent venom.

Reproduction

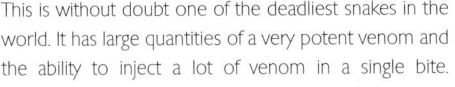

Oviparous, laying 6-17 eggs (63-90 x 29-35 mm) in summer. The young measure 40-60 cm when they hatch and grow rapidly, especially in the first year. Juveniles are perfect replicas of the adults and are deadly venomous. Males often engage in combat, twisting around one another in an attempt to wrestle the weaker male to the ground.

Danger to man

This is without doubt one of the deadliest snakes in the world. It has large quantities of a very potent venom and the ability to inject a lot of venom in a single bite. Because of its length, it may also bite chest-high.

Venom

A very potent neurotoxic venom that is absorbed rapidly. It is responsible primarily for paralysis of nerves, especially those controlling breathing. The victim will experience more and more difficulty in breathing until eventually death results from suffocation. This may take 6-15 hours or much quicker in serious cases. Large quantities of intravenous antivenom may be required to save the victim's life.

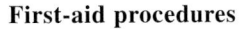

The Black Mamba is so named, not because of its body colour but because of the black inner lining of its mouth.

First-aid procedures

- Immobilise and reassure the patient, who must lie down and be kept as quiet as possible.
- Apply a pressure bandage immediately (see page 9) and immobilise the limb with a splint to reduce the spread of venom.
- Loosen, but do not remove, the bandage if there is severe swelling.
- Transport promptly to hospital.

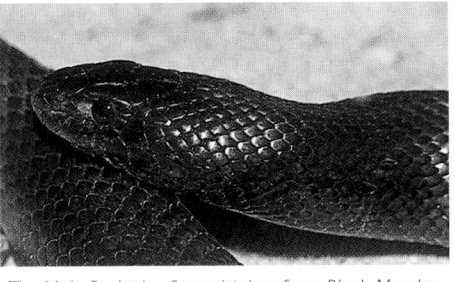

The Mole Snake is often mistaken for a Black Mamba.

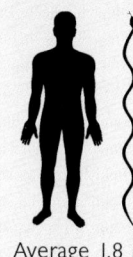

GREEN MAMBA
Dendroaspis angusticeps

Other names
Groenmamba (A)

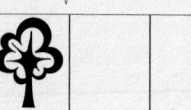

Average 1,8 m
Maximum 2,5 m

LOOK OUT FOR
- Spends most of its time in trees and shrubs.
- Has a light green (not white or yellow) belly.
- Likes to bask in the sun.
- Moves gracefully and effortlessly among the branches of trees.
- Only active in the day.

Preferred habitat
Evergreen lowland forest and moist savanna where it favours bamboo thickets, tea and mango plantations.

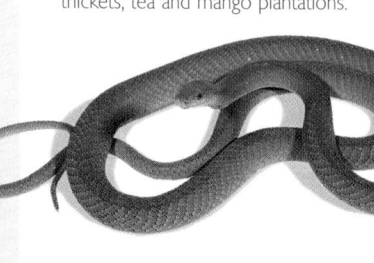

Habits
A tree-living species that seldom ventures to the ground, except to bask or chase its prey. It is active only during daylight hours, and moves gracefully and effortlessly, quickly disappearing into its leafy background. Although an active snake, it is not seen very often. Though shy, it lacks the Black Mamba's nervousness and rarely gapes when threatened. It will, however, strike if provoked. Bites are uncommon.

Similar species
People tend to mistake all green snakes for the Green Mamba. In South Africa, the Green Mamba is only found in coastal forest and does not occur in the Kruger National Park or in the Mpumalanga Province. This snake is often confused with the green variety of the Boomslang and with the harmless Green and Bush snakes of the genus *Philothamnus*. The Green Mamba has a much smaller eye than the Boomslang and a *green belly* as opposed to the white or yellow belly of the Green and Bush snakes. Added to this, the latter snakes are very slender, seldom thicker than a person's smallest finger.

Enemies
Other snakes. Also humans as vast tracts of suitable habitat have been destroyed by developers along the KwaZulu-Natal coast.

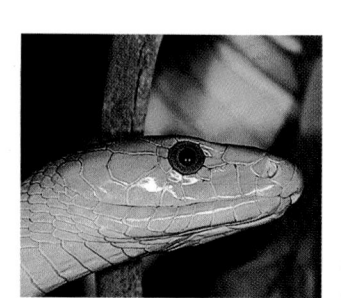

The Green Mamba's head is more slender than that of the Boomslang.

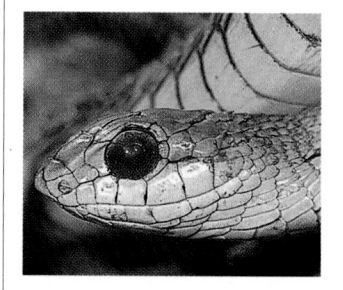

A male Boomslang. Note the enormous eye of this species.

Food and feeding

Its diet consists of birds, their eggs and fledglings as well as small tree-living mammals. Chameleons may be taken by juveniles.

Reproduction

Oviparous, laying 6-17 eggs (47-58 x 25-28 mm) in summer. The eggs are usually deposited in a hollow tree trunk amongst decaying vegetation. Hatchlings measure 35-45 cm in length. Males are known to engage in combat, intertwining their necks and bodies as they push each other onto the ground. Such combat may last several hours. Mating takes place in trees with the tails of both the males and females hanging down.

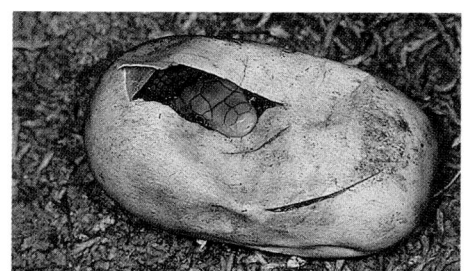

A Green Mamba hatching.

Danger to man

Even though the Green Mamba possesses a deadly venom, it spends most of its life in trees and avoids humans. Bites are rare and are most commonly inflicted on snake handlers.

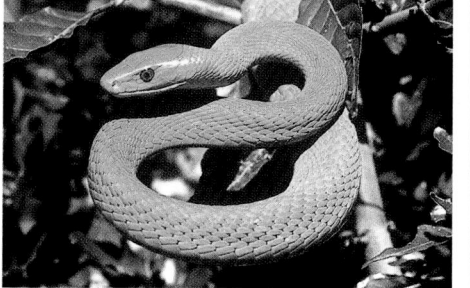

The Green Mamba is a tree-living snake.

The Green Mamba, like the Black Mamba, possesses a potent venom that can easily kill an adult. If given the chance to retreat, however, it will quickly disappear into the closest tree or shrub.

Venom

Dangerously neurotoxic. Similar to that of the Black Mamba but not quite as toxic. It injects smaller quantities of venom than does the Black Mamba. However, its bite is still serious and must be treated as such.

First-aid procedures

- Immobilise and reassure the patient, who must lie down and be kept as quiet as possible.
- Apply a pressure bandage immediately (*see* page 9) and immobilise the limb with a splint to reduce the spread of venom.
- Loosen, but do not remove, the bandage if there is severe swelling.
- Transport promptly to hospital.

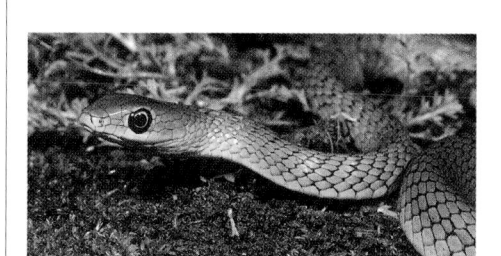

A harmless Green Snake (Philothamnus natalensis).

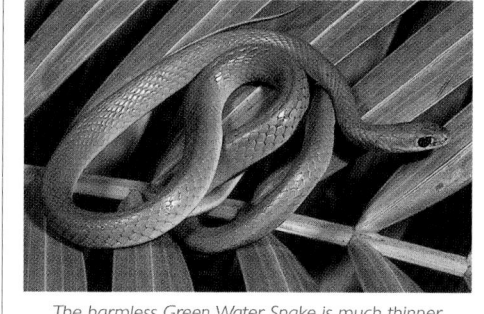

The harmless Green Water Snake is much thinner.

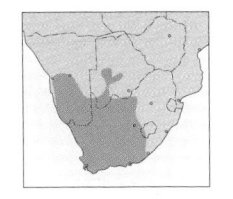

CAPE COBRA
Naja nivea

Other names
Kaapse Kobra, Geel-slang, Koperkapel (A)

Average 1,2 m
Maximum 2 m

LOOK OUT FOR
- Body colour variable, from black to brown, orange, yellow or mottled.
- Stands its ground and spreads a broad hood when confronted.
- Does not *spit* its venom.
- Actiive during the day and early evening.

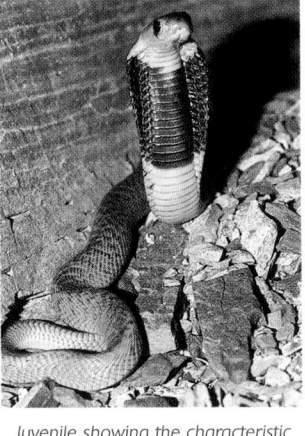

Juvenile showing the characteristic dark markings on the throat.

Preferred habitat
Fynbos, Karoo, arid savanna and Namib Desert where it inhabits rodent burrows, disused termite mounds and rock crevices in arid regions. It is frequently found near human dwellings on farms, especially in the Karoo. Also inhabits partially

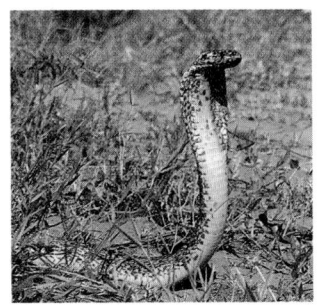

A yellow-speckled Cape Cobra.

developed suburbs and squatter communities where it enters houses to escape the heat of the day.

Restricted largely to the Western, Eastern and Northern Cape; also in the Free State, Botswana and Namibia.

Habits
Active during the day and in the early evenings when it may even climb trees in search of food. When attacked this nervous snake invariably faces its enemy, spreading a broad, impressive hood. It cannot spit its venom. Once on the defensive, it strikes readily. If the aggressor remains motionless, the snake will soon drop to the ground and move off, only to snap back into its defensive pose if it detects movement.

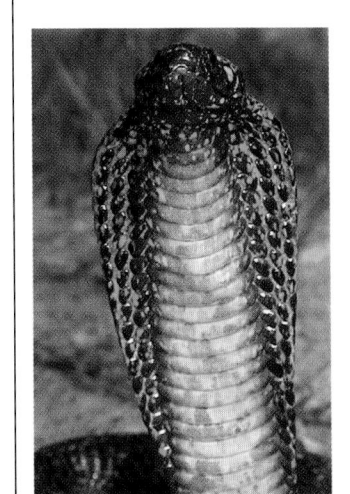

Brown-speckled form, ready to strike.

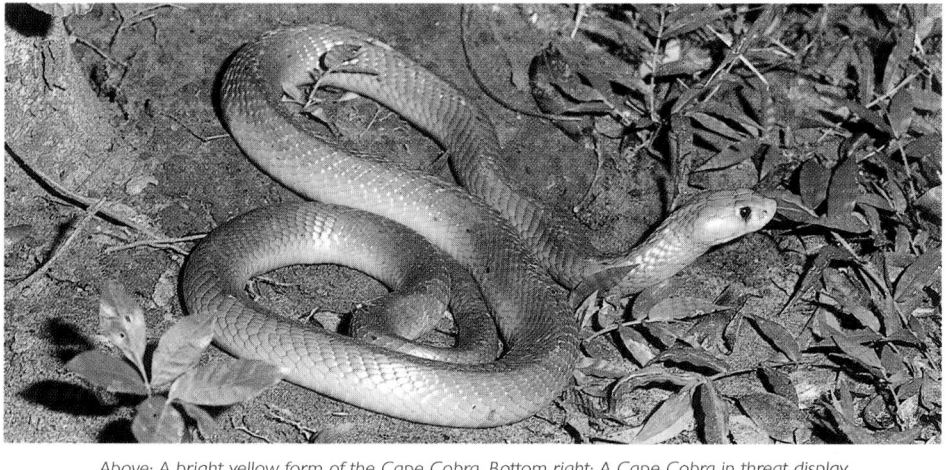

Above: A bright yellow form of the Cape Cobra. Bottom right: A Cape Cobra in threat display.

Similar species

Cape Cobras vary dramatically in colour and may be confused with other cobras and with the Mole Snake.

Enemies

Birds of prey and other snakes.

Cape Cobras often frequent human dwellings, sometimes entering houses. Bites are common and account for most snake-bite fatalities in the Eastern, Northern and Western Cape regions.

Food and feeding

Feeds on rodents, birds, other snakes, lizards and toads. Will climb into trees to reach fledgling birds in their nests and to raid sociable weavers' nests.

Reproduction

Oviparous, laying 8-20 eggs (60-69 x 24-30 mm) in mid-summer. Hatchlings measure 36-40 cm in length.

Danger to man

An extremely dangerous cobra that stands its ground when confronted. Bites are common and often fatal, the victim dying of suffocation.

The harmless Mole Snake, often mistaken for the Cape Cobra, is distinguished by its more pointed snout.

Venom

A highly neurotoxic venom, most potent of any African cobra. As with Black Mamba bites, artificial respiration could keep the victim alive until sufficient quantities of antivenom have been injected.

First-aid procedures

- Immobilise and reassure the patient, who must lie down and be kept as quiet as possible.
- Apply a pressure bandage immediately (*see page 9*) and immobilise the limb with a splint to reduce the spread of venom.
- Loosen, but do not remove, the bandage if there is severe swelling.
- Transport promptly to hospital.

SNOUTED COBRA

Naja annulifera

Other names
Egyptian Cobra (E)
Egiptiese Kobra,
Bosveldkapel (A)

Average 1,2 m
Maximum nearly 3 m

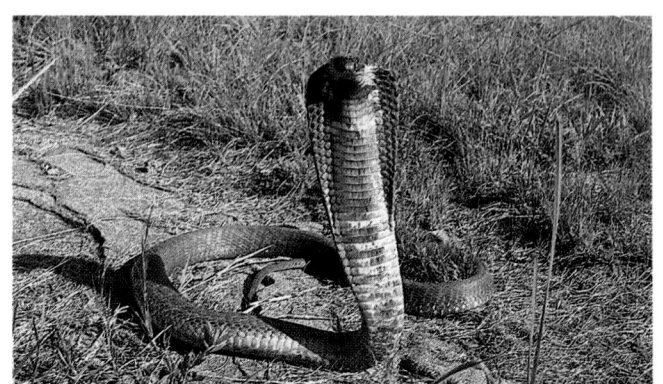

An adult Snouted Cobra in defensive posture, its hood widely spread.

LOOK OUT FOR
- Usually yellowish to greyish-brown, or distinctly barred with 7-11 yellow-brown crossbars on a blue-black background.
- Spreads a wide, impressive hood when cornered.
- Basks in the sun, usually near a safe retreat.
- Usually active from dusk onwards.

Preferred habitat

Arid and moist savanna; common in lowveld and bushveld areas.

Habits

One of Africa's largest cobras, it often occupies a permanent home in a termite mound where it will reside for years if not disturbed. It is active at night, foraging for food from dusk onwards, often venturing into poultry runs. It likes to bask in the morning sun, usually near its retreat into which it will withdraw if disturbed.

It is not an aggressive snake but will assume a formidable posture if cornered. Adults are able to lift as much as half a metre of the body off the ground while spreading a wide, impressive hood. This snake will, however, disappear down the nearest hole or crevice if given the oppor-

tunity. Like the Rinkhals it may pretend to be dead if threatened. It does not spit its venom.

Similar species

May be confused with other cobras including the Forest Cobra and the Cape Cobra (distribution differs), the Black Mamba, the brown variety of the Boomslang, the Mole Snake and some of the larger grass snakes.

> This large cobra is not aggressive and will generally shy away from humans but should be avoided at all costs as it is deadly poisonous.

Enemies

Birds of prey and other snakes.

Food and feeding
Feeds on toads, rodents, birds and their eggs, lizards and other snakes. Often raids poultry runs.

Reproduction
Oviparous, laying 8-33 eggs (47-55 x 25-30 mm) in early summer. The young average 22-34 cm in length.

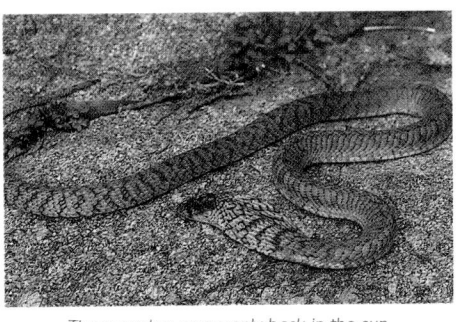
These snakes commonly bask in the sun.

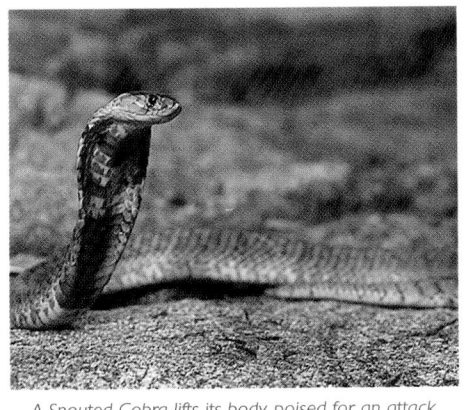
A Snouted Cobra lifts its body, poised for an attack.

Danger to man
A large cobra with a large venom yield. Bites readily when confronted. Large quantities of antivenom may be required in serious cases.

Venom
A potent neurotoxic venom that affects breathing and in untreated cases may cause respiratory failure and death. Initial symptoms often include a burning pain and swelling that may result in blistering. Typically, victims are bitten on the lower leg, and usually at night.

First-aid procedures
- Immobilise and reassure the patient, who must lie down and be kept as quiet as possible.
- Apply a pressure bandage immediately (*see* page 9) and immobilise the limb with a splint to reduce the spread of venom.
- Loosen, but do not remove, the bandage if there is severe swelling.
- Transport promptly to hospital.

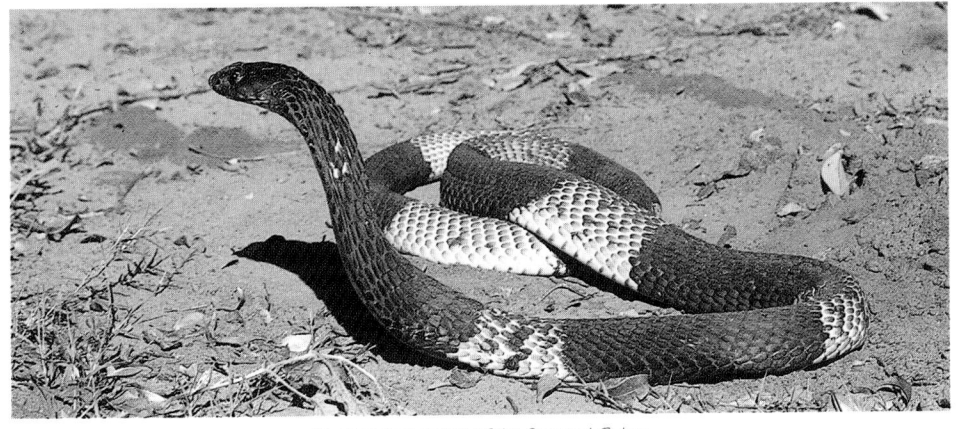
The banded variety of the Snouted Cobra.

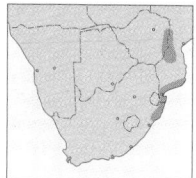

FOREST COBRA
Naja melanoleuca

Other names
Boskobra (A)

Average 1,5 m
Maximum 2,7 m

LOOK OUT FOR
- Highly polished scales which give it a shiny appearance.
- Spreads a narrow hood when cornered.
- Climbs well and is at home in water.
- Prefers thickly vegetated habitats.
- Mainly active at night.

Preferred habitat
Lowland forest and moist savanna where it favours coastal thickets.

Habits
A large cobra normally associated with closed-canopy coastal forest in northern KwaZulu-Natal. It is active and alert, climbs well and is equally at home on land and in water. Though primarily active at night, it likes to bask in the sun. It also forages for food on overcast days. If disturbed, it is quick to disappear into dense thickets, but if cornered will spread a narrow hood and bite readily. Males are known to engage in combat in the mating season. This snake does not *spit* its venom.

This is a very large cobra that avoids humans but bites readily when cornered.

Similar species
Often mistaken for the Black Mamba but distinguished by its highly polished scales, which give it a shiny appearance. May also be mistaken for some of the larger grass snakes.

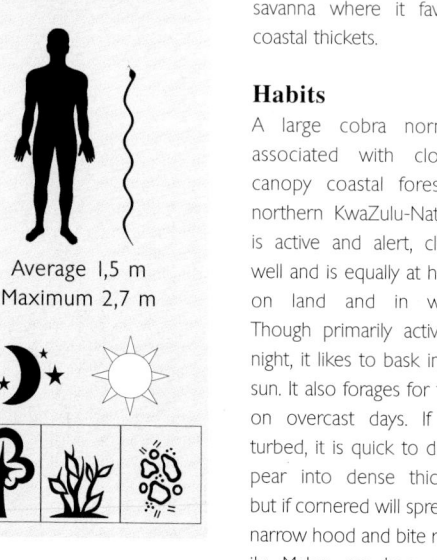

The Forest Cobra has highly polished scales.

Enemies
Other snakes.

Food and feeding
Feeds on toads, frogs, small mammals, birds and snakes. Also feeds on fish.

Reproduction
Oviparous, laying 11-26 smooth white eggs in summer (46-61 × 24-32 mm) that stick together in a bunch. The young measure 27-38 cm in length.

Danger to man

Though extremely venomous, this retiring snake seldom features in snake-bite accidents.

Venom

Potently neurotoxic but because of this snake's restricted distribution and shy nature, bites are virtually unheard of in South Africa.

First-aid procedures

- Immobilise and reassure the patient, who must lie down and be kept as quiet as possible.
- Apply a pressure bandage immediately (*see* page 9) and immobilise the limb with a splint to reduce the spread of venom.
- Loosen, but do not remove, the bandage if there is severe swelling.
- Transport promptly to hospital.

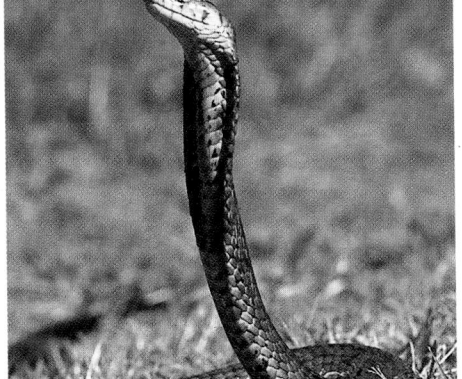

A Forest Cobra in a defensive pose.

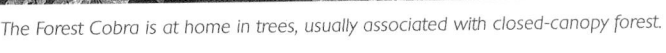

The Forest Cobra is at home in trees, usually associated with closed-canopy forest.

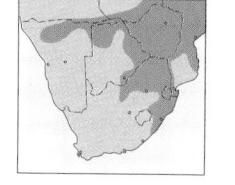

MOZAMBIQUE SPITTING COBRA

Naja mossambica 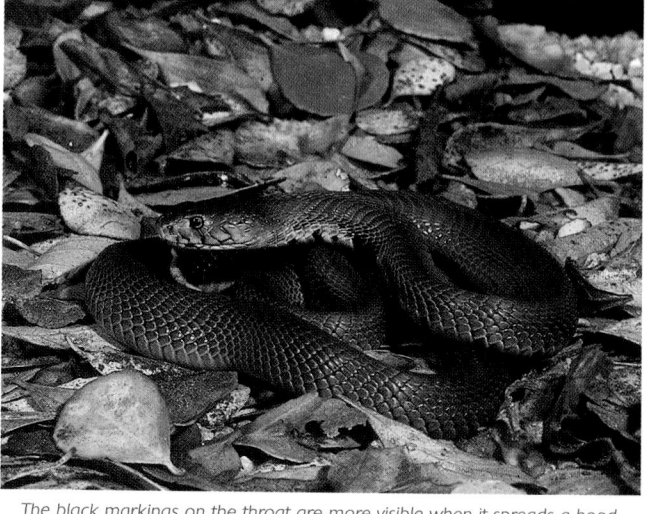 VERY DANGEROUS

Other names
Mosambiekse
Spoegkobra (A);
M'fezi (Zulu)

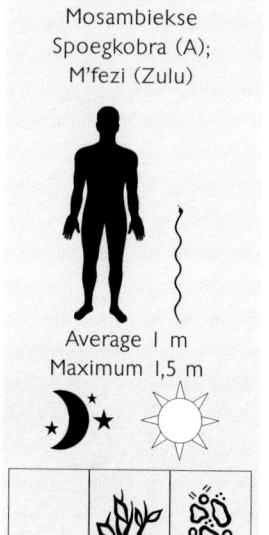

Average 1 m
Maximum 1,5 m

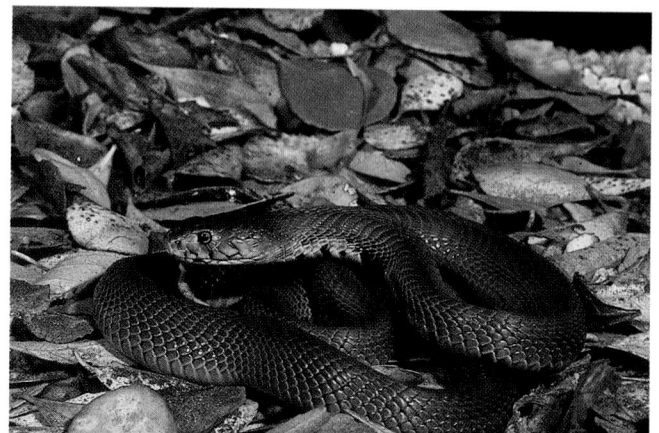

The black markings on the throat are more visible when it spreads a hood.

LOOK OUT FOR
- Slate-grey to olive-brown above with black bars or blotches on the throat – clearly visible when it spreads a hood.
- Forms a hood when threatened.
- May *spit* its venom.
- Adults active by night; juveniles active by day.

Preferred habitat
The most common of the region's cobras, found largely in moist savanna and lowland forest where it favours broken rocky country, hollow trees, termite mounds and animal holes, often close to permanent water.

Habits
May bask near a retreat or forage on overcast days, otherwise it is more active at night. Juveniles, on the other hand, are quite active in the day. It is a shy, retiring snake that seldom stands its ground. If cornered it may spread a narrow hood, but will not hold the pose for long. Its main defence, other than going into hiding, is to eject or spit its venom.

The fangs are specially modified for spitting: the venom canal openings at the tips are directed forwards and at right angles to the fangs, enabling the snake to eject its venom to a distance greater than two metres. This snake does not always spread a hood before spitting and may only open its mouth slightly before doing so. It can spit effectively from a concealed position within a rock crevice. The venom supply is seemingly inexhaustible. If venom lands on the hair, face or arms it poses no threat, but in the eyes it causes an immediate burning sensation and should be washed out immediately with large quantities of water or any other bland liquid (*see* 'Spitting Snakes' on page 10).

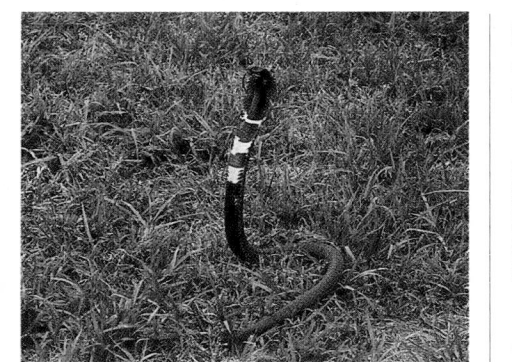

The Rinkhals (above) is often confused with this species.

Similar species

May be confused with other cobras, the Mole Snake and the Rinkhals.

Enemies

Preyed upon by snakes.

Food and feeding

Preys on toads, small mammals, birds, lizards, insects and snakes. May be found in poultry runs and in the vicinity of houses in search of food.

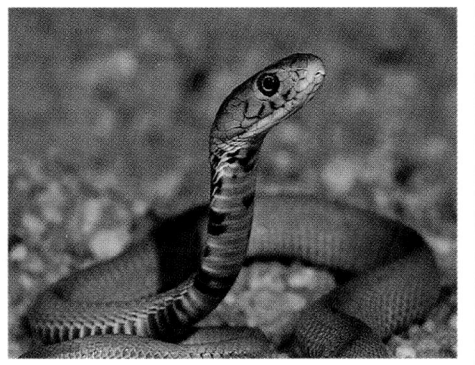

A juvenile poised to spit venom.

Reproduction

Oviparous, laying 10-22 eggs (35 × 20 mm) in mid-summer. Hatchlings measure 23-25 cm in length.

Danger to man

A common snake with a potent venom. Accounts for many bites in KwaZulu-Natal and Mpumalanga.

> This dangerous snake is very common and often forages around houses at night. Beware of it spitting venom – which may enter the eyes.

Venom

Predominantly cytotoxic, causing serious local tissue damage that often requires skin grafts. Only slight neurotoxic symptoms, such as drowsiness, may occur and fatalities are rare. The early administration of antivenom may reduce the extent of tissue damage.

For treatment of venom in the eyes, see 'Spitting Snakes' on page 10.

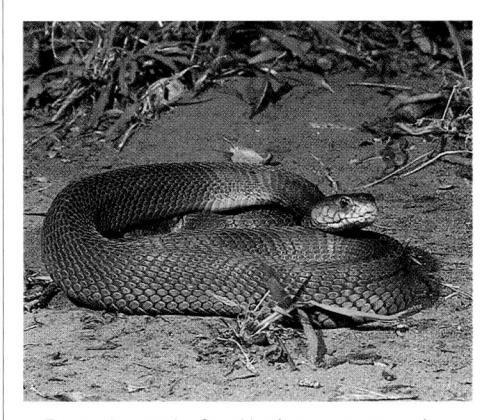

This snake may be found basking on overcast days.

First-aid procedures

▦ Immobilise and reassure the patient, who must lie down and be kept as quiet as possible.

▦ Apply a pressure bandage immediately (see page 9) and immobilise the limb with a splint to reduce the spread of venom.

▦ Loosen, but do not remove, the bandage if there is severe swelling.

▦ Transport promptly to hospital.

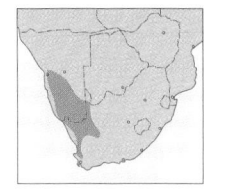

BLACK SPITTING COBRA

Naja nigricollis woodi

Other names
Swartspoegslang;
Swart Spoegkobra (A)

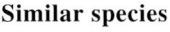

Average 1,2 m
Maximum 2 m

LOOK OUT FOR
- Uniform black above and below.
- Juveniles greyish with a black head.
- Spreads a hood when threatened and *spits* large quantities of venom.

Preferred habitat
Mountains and rocky outcrops as well as dry, rocky watercourses in the Namib Desert and Karoo.

Habits
A rare snake that for many years was thought to be a black variety of the Cape Cobra. Often seen on the road at Aninauspas between Port Nolloth and Steinkopf. The Black Spitting Cobra spits venom in the same way as does the Mozambique Spitting Cobra but appears to be more effective, ejecting large quantities of venom at a time.

Similar species
Often confused with dark varieties of the Cape Cobra. May also be confused with dark varieties of the Mole Snake.

Enemies
Preyed upon by other snakes.

Food and feeding
Feeds on snakes, lizards, toads and small mammals.

Reproduction
Oviparous, laying 10-20 eggs.

Danger to man
Possesses a very potent venom but is seldom encountered by man. This snake is listed as rare in the latest *South African Red Data Book – Reptiles and Amphibians*.

The Black Spitting Cobra

A prolific 'spitter' that ejects large quantities of venom when cornered or threatened.

Venom
Potently cytotoxic, causing severe tissue damage.

For the treatment of venom entering the eyes, *see* 'Spitting Snakes' on page 10.

38

Did you know?

Not all snakes spit. In fact, only four spitting snakes are found in southern Africa: the Mozambique Spitting Cobra and the Rinkhals, and the less common Black Spitting Cobra and Western Barred Spitting Cobra. These snakes have the ability to eject their venom over a distance of about two metres. In the eyes of a potential predator, the venom causes temporary blindness and great discomfort, giving the snake time to escape. When biting, these snakes inject the same venom that they spit. Spitting snakes have a seemingly inexhaustible supply of venom and after spitting several times still possess sufficient venom to kill someone.

The Rinkhals always spits from an upright or reared position while exposing a hood. Once reared, it draws its head backwards and, while lunging forward, sprays two rows of venom towards any form of danger. The Mozambique Spitting Cobra spits its venom from virtually any position, even when concealed in a rock crevice!

First-aid procedures

- Immobilise and reassure the patient, who must lie down and be kept as quiet as possible.
- Apply a pressure bandage immediately (*see* page 9) and immobilise the limb with a splint to reduce the spread of venom.
- Loosen, but do not remove, the bandage if there is severe swelling.
- Transport promptly to hospital.

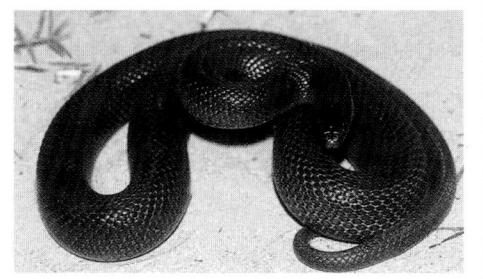

The similar but harmless Mole Snake.

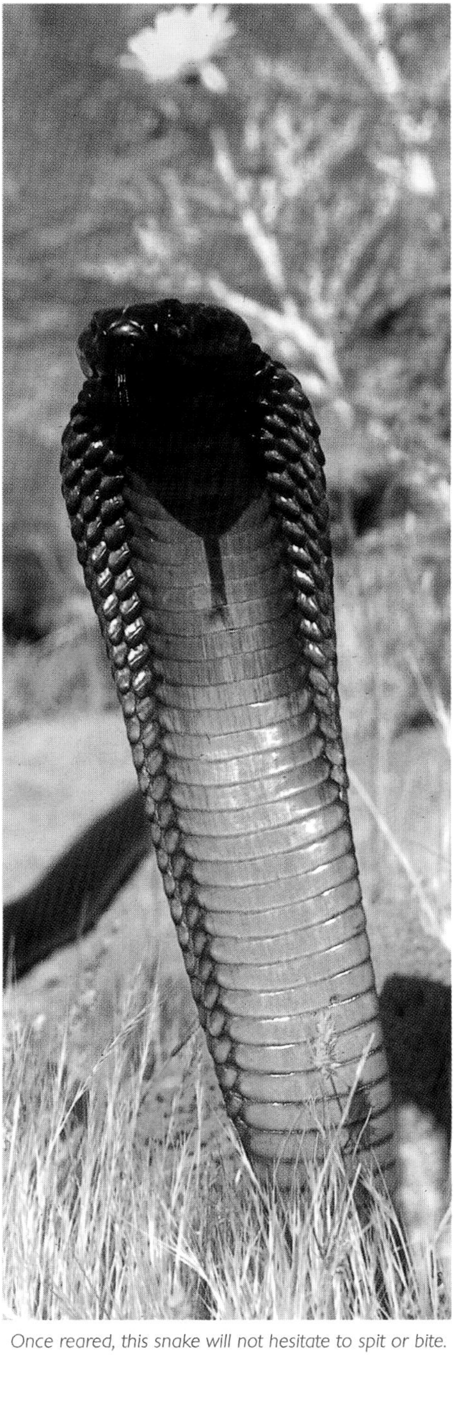

Once reared, this snake will not hesitate to spit or bite.

WESTERN BARRED SPITTING COBRA

Naja nigricollis nigricincta

Other names
Zebra Snake (E);
Sebraslang (A)

Average 1 m
Maximum 1,5 m

Preferred habitat
The Namib Desert and Karoo regions of central and northern Namibia, extending into the southern reaches of Angola.

Habits
A nocturnal snake that is often found on tarred roads. It is shy, choosing to escape if it has the choice, but if cornered will spread a hood and may spit its venom.

Similar species
May be confused with the harmless Tiger Snake and the Coral Snake.

Enemies
Predatory birds and snakes. Vehicles on tarred roads kill many individuals.

Food and feeding
Feeds on other snakes, lizards, toads and small mammals.

Reproduction
Oviparous, laying 10-22 eggs.

> This snake spits readily and effectively but is not confrontational and usually chooses to escape.

Danger to man
Common where it occurs, and accounting for many bites among humans. This snake's venom is dangerously cytotoxic.

LOOK OUT FOR
- Distinct black rings or crossbars on the body and tail.
- Often found on tarred roads.
- Active at night, especially after rain.

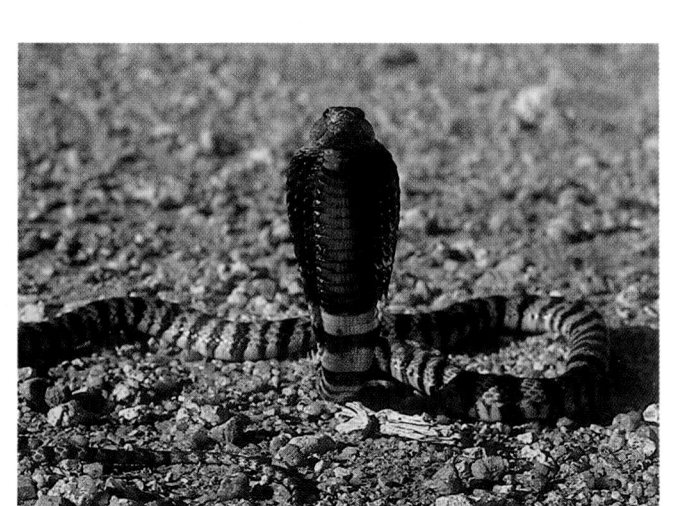

The Western Barred Spitting Cobra in defensive pose, ready to spit or bite.

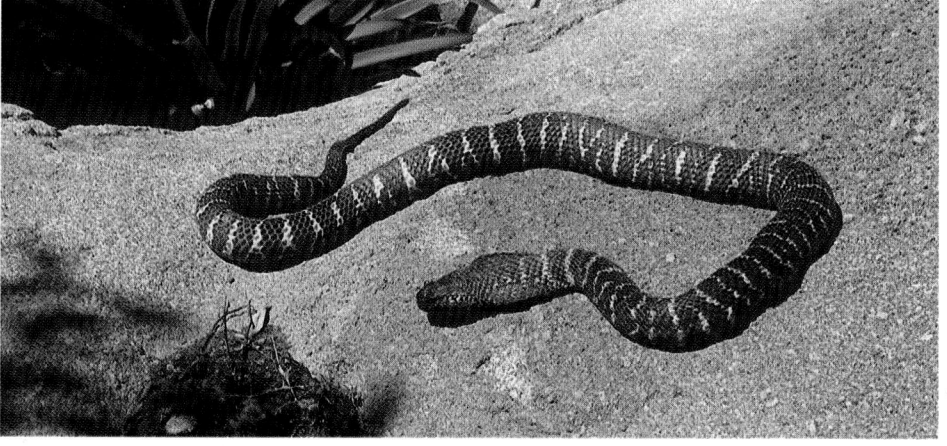
A Western Barred Spitting Cobra sunning itself.

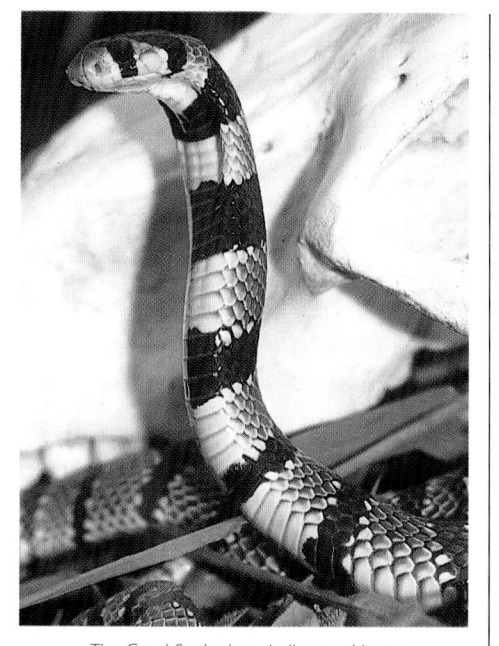
The Coral Snake has similar markings.

The mildly venomous Tiger Snake is also similar. Below: Western Barred Spitting Cobra ready to spit.

Venom

A potent cytotoxic venom which may cause severe tissue damage. It bites and also spits venom. For treatment of venom in the eyes, *see* 'Spitting Snakes' on page 10.

First-aid procedures

- Immobilise and reassure the patient, who must lie down and be kept as quiet as possible.
- Apply a pressure bandage immediately (*see* page 9) and immobilise the limb with a splint to reduce the spread of venom.
- Loosen, but do not remove, the bandage if there is severe swelling.
- Transport promptly to hospital.

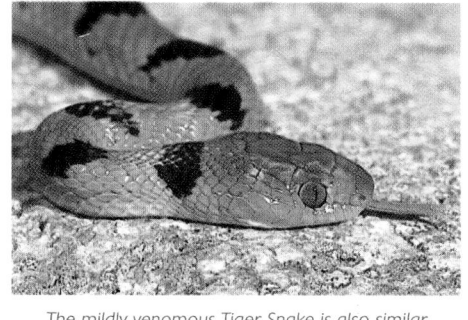

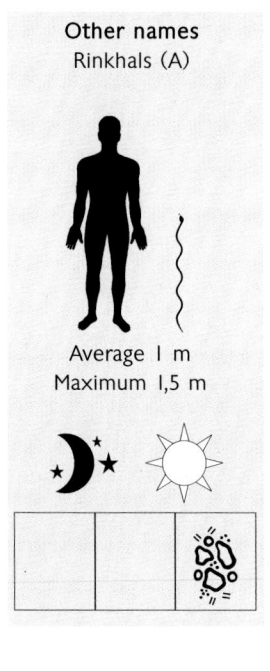

RINKHALS

Hemachatus haemachatus

Other names

Rinkhals (A)

Average I m
Maximum I,5 m

Preferred habitat

Grassland, moist savanna, lowland forest and fynbos; often encountered on smallholdings in and around Johannesburg.

Habits

Common throughout most of its range, especially the grasslands of the higher-lying areas. In spite of urban development, it is still common around Johannesburg, especially near vleis, dams, compost heaps, stables and rockeries.

> This common, venomous snake frequents human dwellings, often entering houses.

Though mainly active at night, it basks frequently and may venture into houses by day. The Rinkhals disappears quickly when disturbed, unless cornered when it will lift as much as half its body off the ground with its hood spread and the two or three white bars on the throat clearly visible.

Like the Mozambique Spitting Cobra it *spits* its venom but always from a reared position. When spitting it throws the raised part of its body forward, often hissing at the same time. It spits effectively up to two to three metres, not aiming accurately but rather spraying the venom in the direction of its opponent.

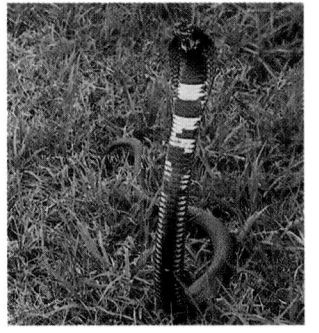

A typical Highveld colour form.

If approached closely, the Rinkhals may drop to the ground, twist the anterior portion of the body sideways or upside down, and *play dead*. The tongue is often left hanging out of a partially opened mouth. If it is picked up while playing dead, it may hang limply, but could equally strike out at any time.

Bites by this snake are rare and are more often inflicted on dogs and horses. Despite its cobra-like appearance, the Rinkhals is not a true cobra. It has keeled dorsal scales, gives birth to live young (true cobras lay eggs) and there are also some important skeletal differences between this snake and cobras.

Similar species

May be confused with the Mole Snake. In many areas farmers incorrectly refer to the Mozambique Spitting Cobra and the Snouted Cobra as the Rinkhals.

Enemies

Predatory birds and other snakes. Bullfrogs also eat the young. Development appears to be this snake's biggest threat as more and more habitat is destroyed.

Food and feeding

Very partial to toads but also feeds on lizards, rodents, snakes, birds and their eggs. Eggs are swallowed whole.

Reproduction

Viviparous, giving birth to 20-30 young, but as many as 60 in late summer. The young, averaging 18 cm in length, are perfect replicas of the adults.

Danger to man

Although this snake's venom is potentially deadly, it is not as potent as that of most cobras. Human fatalities are rare.

Venom

A dangerous neurotoxic venom that affects breathing and, in untreated cases, may cause respiratory failure and death. Antivenom is effective against this snake's venom. Bites are rare and fatalities virtually unheard of.

For treatment of venom in the eyes, *see* 'Spitting Snakes on page 10.

Did you know?

Most venomous snakes have full control over their venom glands and will often bite without injecting any venom. Harmless snakes have neither fangs nor venom glands, but many have the ability to bite and draw blood.

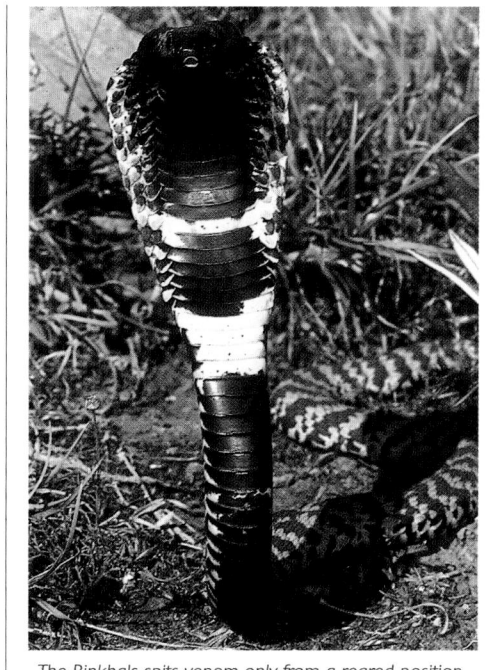

The Rinkhals spits venom only from a reared position.

First-aid procedures

- Immobilise and reassure the patient, who must lie down and be kept as quiet as possible.
- Apply a pressure bandage immediately (*see* page 9) and immobilise the limb with a splint to reduce the spread of venom.
- Loosen, but do not remove, the bandage if there is severe swelling.
- Transport promptly to hospital.

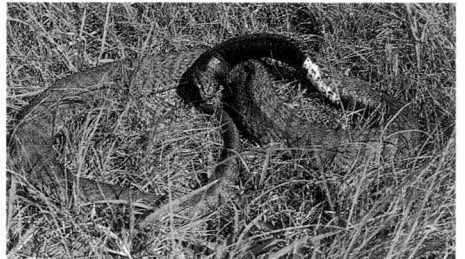

A Rinkhals playing dead.

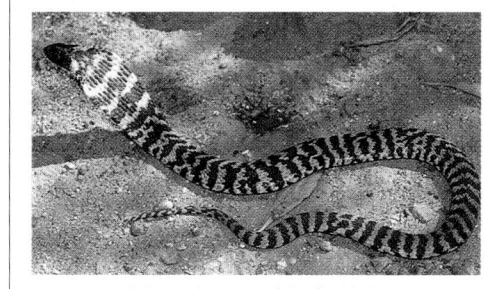

A barred variety of the Rinkhals.

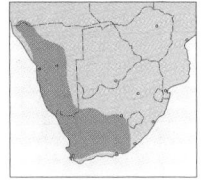

CORAL SNAKE

Aspidelaps lubricus

Other names
Koraalslang (A)

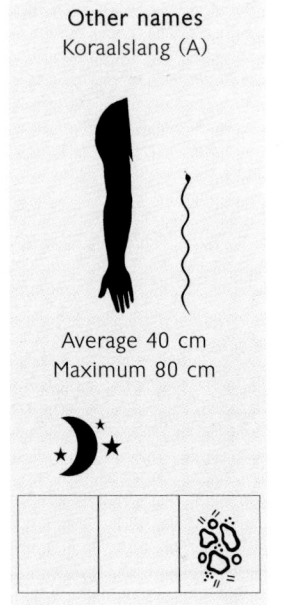

Average 40 cm
Maximum 80 cm

Preferred habitat
Rocky outcrops, stony and dry sandy regions in the Namib Desert, arid savanna, Karoo and fynbos.

Habits
Spends much of its life underground, emerging at night to forage for food. Very active after rains, when many individuals are killed on roads by vehicles. It is a bad-tempered snake that spreads a narrow hood when cornered. It will strike repeatedly while hissing and lunging forward.

Similar species
The Tiger Snake and the Western Barred Spitting Cobra.

Enemies
Snakes and birds of prey.

Food and feeding
Feeds on lizards, small snakes and rodents.

Reproduction
Oviparous, laying 3-11 eggs (45-54 × 14-25 mm) in the summer months. The young measure from 17-18 cm in length.

> When cornered, this snake will strike repeatedly, hissing and lunging forward at the same time.

LOOK OUT FOR
- Several black cross-bars down the length of its body.
- Specimens from Namibia have a distinct black head.
- Lifts its head off the ground and spreads a narrow hood.
- Strikes repeatedly while hissing and lunging forward.
- Active at night.

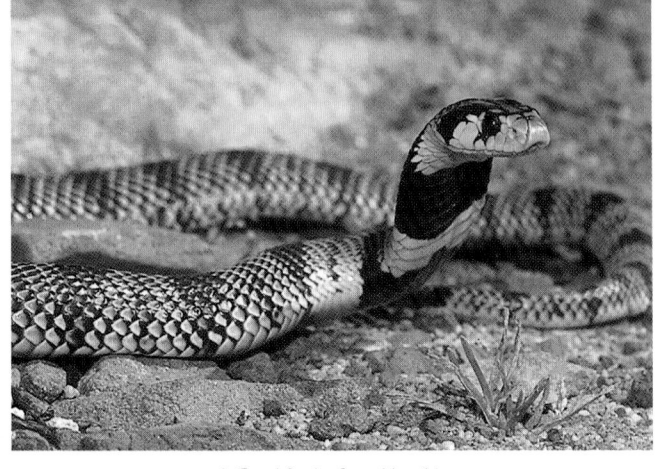

A Coral Snake from Namibia.

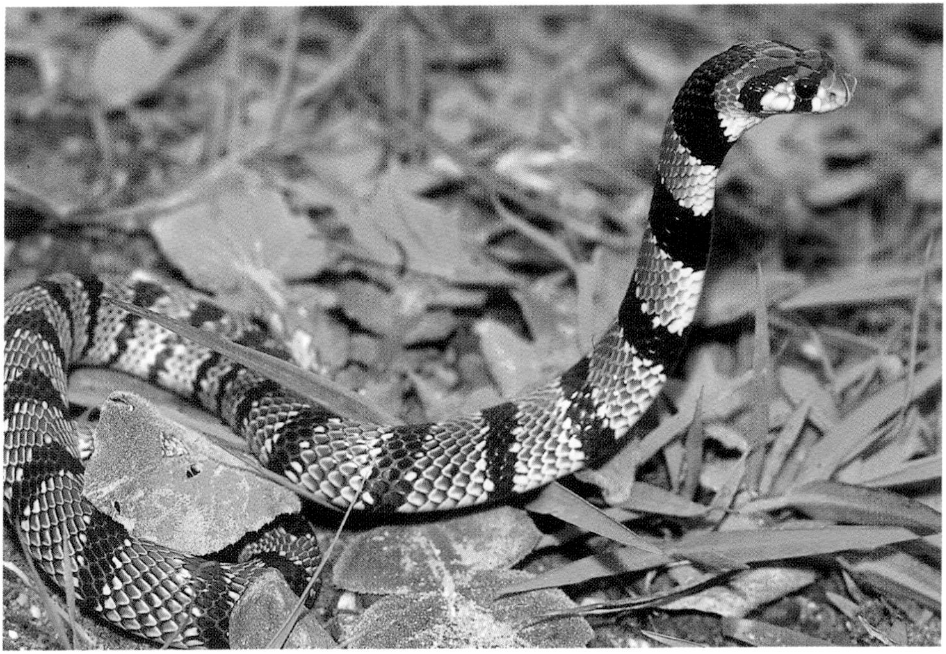

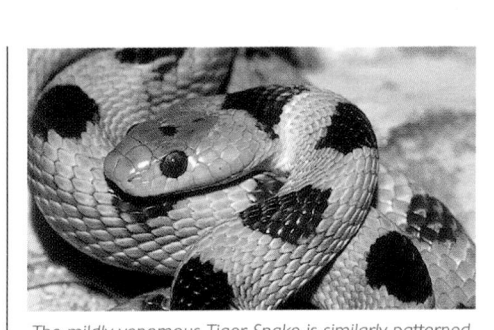

The Coral Snake is nocturnal and emerges at night to forage; it is also very active after rains.

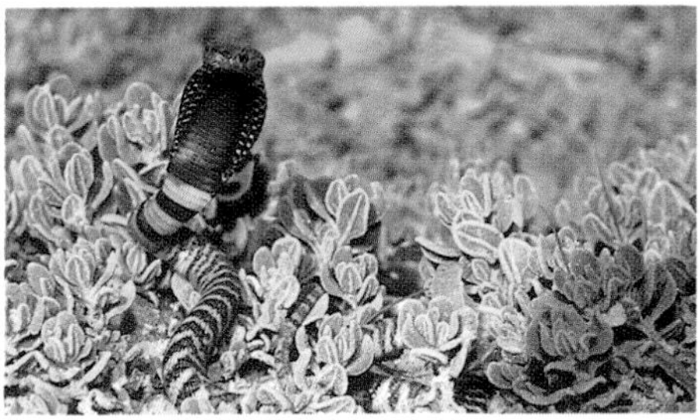

The similar Western Barred Spitting Cobra.

The mildly venomous Tiger Snake is similarly patterned.

Danger to man

Bites from this snake in South Africa have not resulted in life-threatening symptoms but in Namibia this snake has reportedly killed two children.

Venom

Very little is known about this snake's venom but it is believed to be dangerously neurotoxic, and victims must be treated promptly.

First-aid procedures

- Immobilise and reassure the patient, who must lie down and be kept as quiet as possible.
- Apply a pressure bandage immediately (*see* page 9) and immobilise the limb with a splint to reduce the spread of venom.
- Loosen, but do not remove, the bandage if there is severe swelling.
- Transport promptly to hospital.

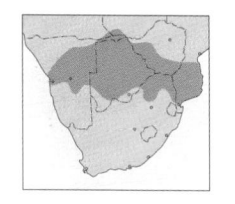

SHIELD-NOSE SNAKE

Aspidelaps scutatus

Other names
Skildneusslang (A)

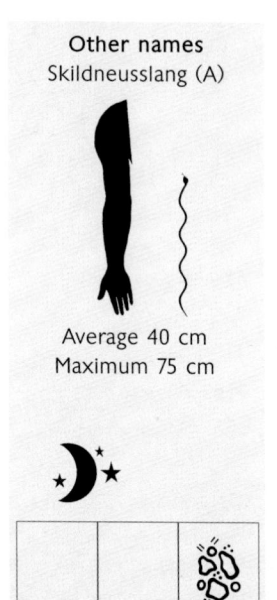

Average 40 cm
Maximum 75 cm

LOOK OUT FOR
- A series of brown blotches on the back.
- White markings in the throat region.
- A snout covered with a large rostral scale.
- May play dead.
- Active at night.

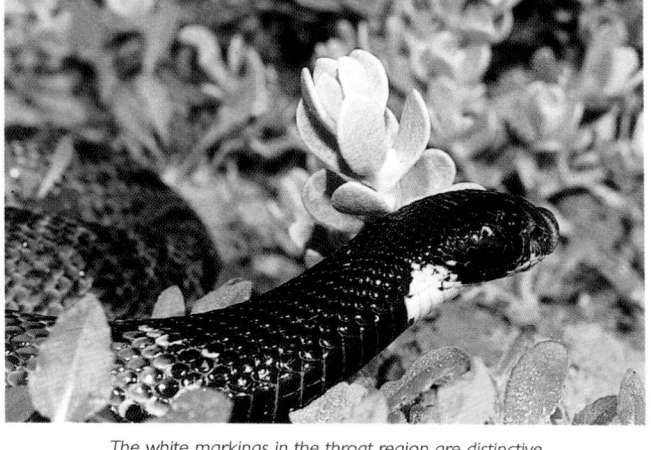

The white markings in the throat region are distinctive.

Preferred habitat
Sandy and stony regions in the Namib Desert, and moist and arid savannna.

Habits
Hides during the day and forages for food at night. This snake has a large rostral scale, which it uses as a bulldozer to push through sandy soil. It may play dead, like the Rinkhals, but when molested it performs like a Coral Snake, raising its head while hissing and striking repeatedly. It does not spread a hood.

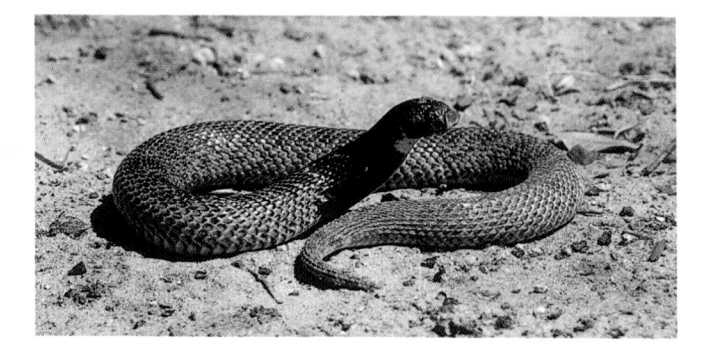

A Shield-nose Snake from Hoedspruit in Mpumalanga.

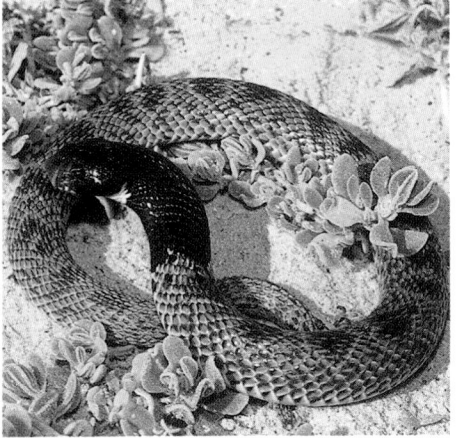

The Shield-nose Snake usually hides during the day.

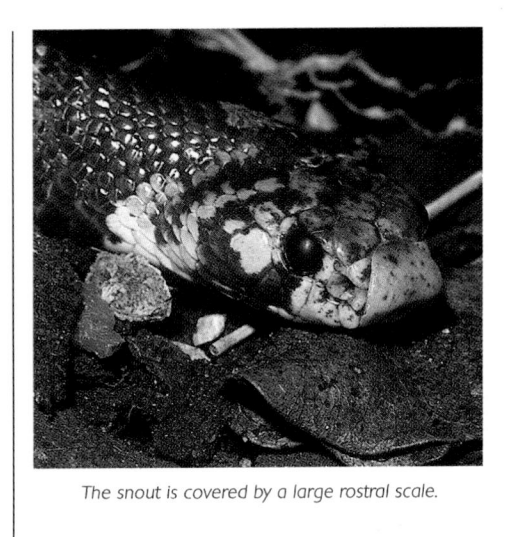

The snout is covered by a large rostral scale.

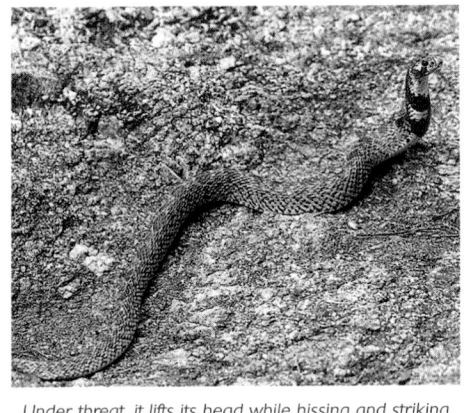

Under threat, it lifts its head while hissing and striking.

Similar species
May be confused with the Tiger Snake or the Western Barred Spitting Cobra.

Enemies
Other snakes.

Food and feeding
Eats small mammals, amphibians, lizards and snakes.

Reproduction
Oviparous, laying 4-14 eggs.

Danger to man
Bites from this snake seldom result in serious symptoms but at least one death has been reported.

Venom
Little is known of this snake's venom. Mild neurological symptoms may result such as slurred speech, drooping eyelids and partial paralysis accompanied by much pain. In some cases symptoms have included severe pain and swelling with no neurological symptoms whatsoever. The symptoms may persist for several days.

> When threatened, the Shield-nose Snake will lift its head off the ground and strike repeatedly, hissing at the same time.

First-aid procedures
- Immobilise and reassure the patient, who must lie down and be kept as quiet as possible.
- Apply a pressure bandage immediately (see page 9) and immobilise the limb with a splint to reduce the spread of venom.
- Loosen, but do not remove, the bandage if there is severe swelling.
- Transport promptly to hospital.

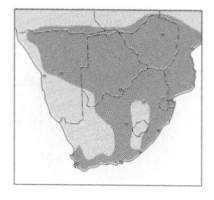

BOOMSLANG

Dispholidus typus

Other names
Boomslang (A)

Average 1,2 m
Maximum 2 m

LOOK OUT FOR
- Usually in trees.
- Enormous eyes and a short stubby head.
- Colour variable: juveniles (less than 40 cm) usually grey with huge emerald eyes. Adult females usually brown. Males bright green, sometimes with black-edged scales. Brick-red specimens found in some areas.

Preferred habitat
Trees and shrubs in arid and moist savanna, lowland forest and fynbos.

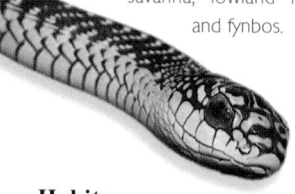

Habits
A shy diurnal snake that spends most of its time in trees and shrubs. It may descend to the ground to bask or hunt for food, but is quick to disappear into the leafy concealment of the closest tree when disturbed. It is extremely well camouflaged and very difficult to detect.

The Boomslang actively hunts for food during the day and mostly in trees. When food is spotted, it freezes, moves its head from side to side and then swoops onto its prey, holding it firmly in its jaws while the fangs move with a chewing motion.

When provoked the Boomslang will inflate its neck to twice its normal size, exposing the bright skin between the scales. In this state, it will not hesitate to strike and will do so with jerky movements. However, very few people have been bitten by the Boomslang.

It is a popular fallacy that the Boomslang, being back fanged, cannot easily bite and must get hold of one's finger to inject venom. This snake, like many others, can open its mouth as wide as 170 degrees.

Similar species
Often confused with the Black and Green mambas and with the harmless green snakes of the genus *Philothamnus*.

Enemies
Predatory birds and other snakes. Birds such as bulbuls often mob it.

Food and feeding
Actively hunts chameleons and other tree-living lizards, birds, nestlings, eggs (swallowed whole) and frogs. Small mammals are seldom taken.

Reproduction
Oviparous, laying 8-14 or as many as 27 eggs (27-53 × 18-37mm) in late spring to mid-summer. The young measure 29-38 cm.

Danger to man
Though deadly venomous, this shy snake very seldom bites. Most victims have been snake handlers and park attendants.

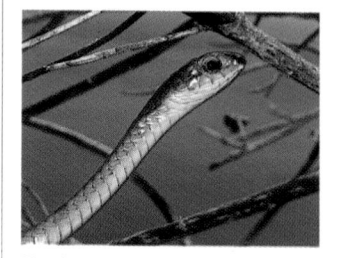

The female is usually brown in colour.
Top: The male Boomslang.

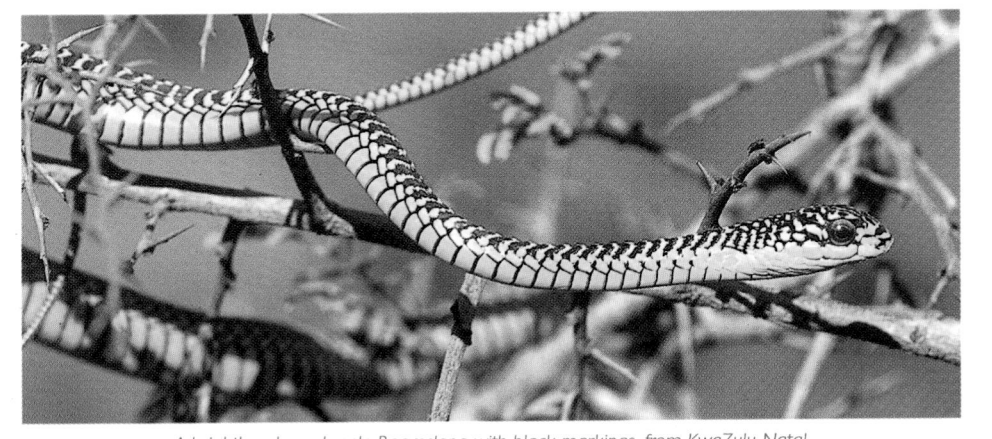

A brightly coloured male Boomslang with black markings, from KwaZulu-Natal.

Venom

Potently haemotoxic, causing severe bleeding internally and from the mucous surfaces. May result in fatal haemorrhage if untreated. Although the venom is extremely potent it is slow-acting and may take more than 24-48 hours to produce serious symptoms. An effective Boomslang antivenom is available from the South African Institute of Medical Research in Johannesburg. Victims should be hospitalised for at least 48 hours.

First-aid procedures

- Immobilise and reassure the patient, who must lie down and be kept as quiet as possible.
- Apply a pressure bandage immediately (*see* page 9) and immobilise the limb with a splint to reduce the spread of venom.
- Loosen, but do not remove, the bandage if there is severe swelling.
- Transport promptly to hospital.

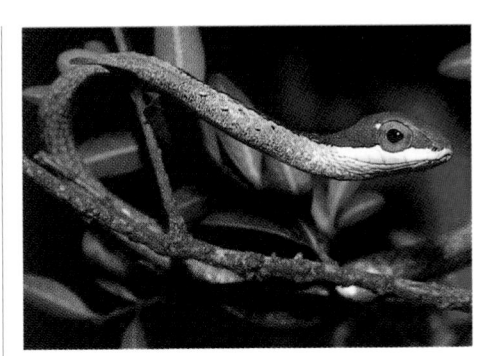

The juvenile has very large emerald eyes.

The chances of being bitten by this snake are extremely remote unless one actually handles it. Never handle any small snakes, especially if brought into the house by a cat.

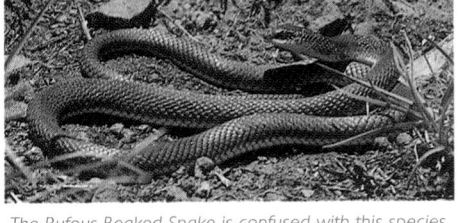

The Rufous Beaked Snake is confused with this species.

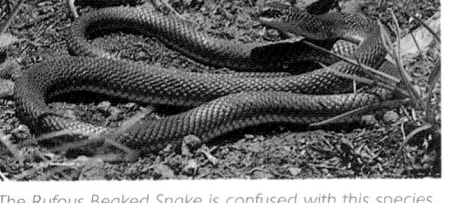

The similar but harmless Green Snake, KwaZulu-Natal.

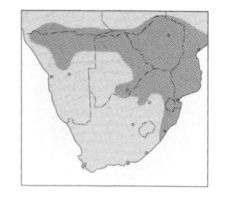

TWIG SNAKE

Thelotornis capensis

Other names
Vine Snake;
Bird Snake (E);
Voëlslang (A)

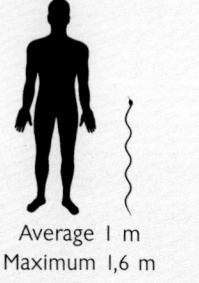

Average 1 m
Maximum 1,6 m

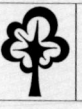 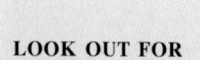

Preferred habitat
Trees and shrubs in moist savanna and lowland forest.

Habits
A slender, mostly tree-living snake that prefers low shrubs, bushes and trees where its cryptic coloration blends so well with the background that it is seldom seen. It moves gracefully and swiftly when disturbed.

Though timid and retiring, it will inflate its neck to display the bright skin between the scales when threatened. This is usually followed by lunging strikes while the bright tongue flickers in a wavy motion.

It actively hunts for food during the day, first approaching its prey in short spurts, then darting forward to seize its prey. The prey is held firmly in the jaws while the venom takes effect.

Males engage in combat, intertwining their bodies while attempting to push one another's heads down.

Though timid by nature, this snake may react viciously if handled.

Similar species
Some of the grass or sand snakes. Twig Snakes, however, are usually found in shrubs and trees.

Enemies
Birds of prey and other snakes.

Food and feeding
Largely chameleons and other tree-dwelling lizards. Also takes small mammals, fledgling birds and other snakes.

LOOK OUT FOR
- Usually found in trees and shrubs.
- Perfectly camouflaged.
- Has a keyhole-shaped pupil.
- Has a bright red and black tongue, which flickers regularly.

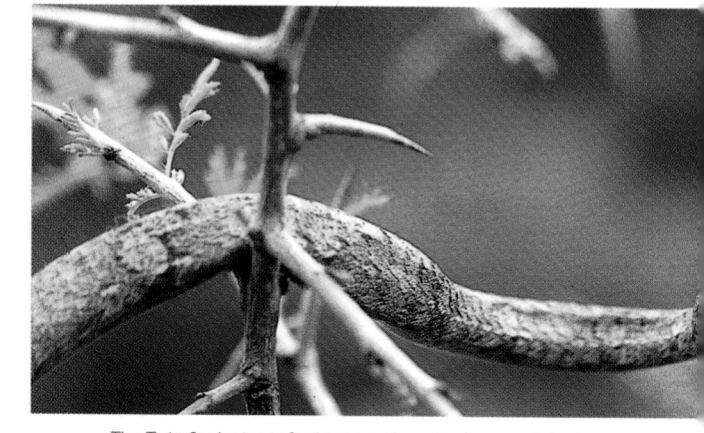

The Twig Snake is perfectly camouflaged in trees and shrubs.

Reproduction
Oviparous, laying 4-18 eggs (25-41 × 13-17 mm) in summer. The young measure 23-33 cm in length.

Danger to man
Like the Boomslang, the Twig Snake is very shy and the chance of being bitten by it is very slight.

Venom
Dangerously haemotoxic and very similar in effect to the venom of the Boomslang. Bites are rare, which is fortunate because at present there is no antivenom

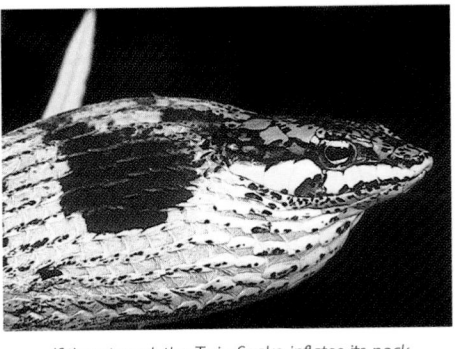

If threatened, the Twig Snake inflates its neck and will not hesitate to strike.

against the venom of the Twig Snake; the monovalent Boomslang antivenom does not neutralise the venom of this snake. Victims must be hospitalised as soon as possible. Human fatalities are rare.

First-aid procedures
- Immobilise and reassure the patient, who must lie down and be kept as quiet as possible.
- Apply a pressure bandage immediately (*see* page 9) and immobilise the limb with a splint to reduce the spread of venom.
- Loosen, but do not remove, the bandage if there is severe swelling.
- Transport promptly to hospital.

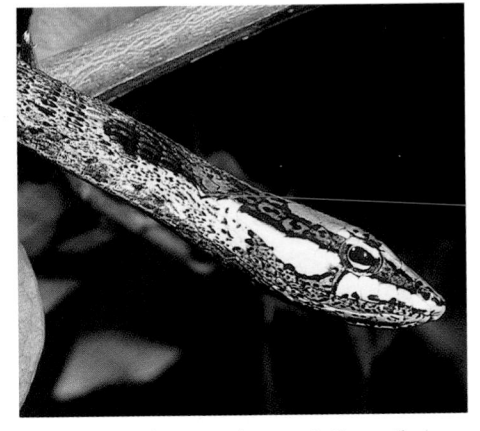

The Twig Snake has unusual eyes; note the pupil's shape.

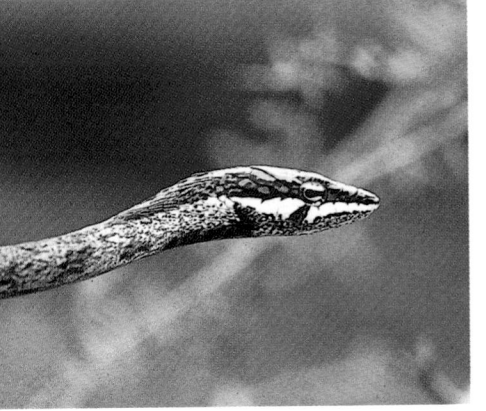

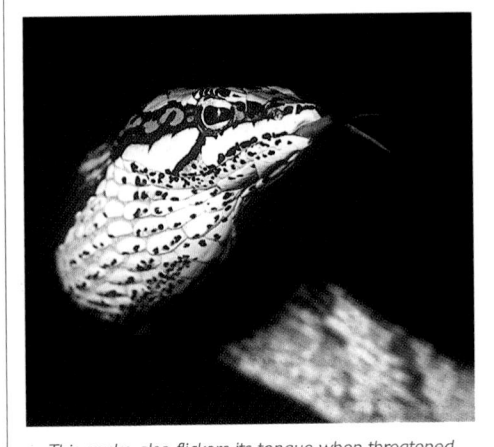

This snake also flickers its tongue when threatened.

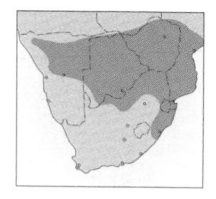

STILETTO SNAKE

Atractaspis bibronii

Other names
Southern or Bibron's
Burrowing Asp (E)
Suidelike Sypikslang (A)

Average 30 cm
Maximum 70 cm

The eyes of this snake are reduced as it spends most of its time underground.

LOOK OUT FOR
- A uniform purple-brown to black colour above.
- Pointed head indistinct from the rest of the body.
- Tail ends in a sharp spike.
- Emerges after heavy rain.
- Usually nocturnal.

Preferred habitat

A burrowing species usually found in deserted termite mounds, under rotting logs or beneath sun-warmed rocks in lowland forest, and both moist and arid savanna.

Habits

Previously called the Mole Adder or Burrowing Adder, this nocturnal snake usually emerges on warm wet summer evenings, especially after heavy rains. Individuals are often exposed during excavations. It is an extremely irascible snake that bites readily. The fangs are positioned horizontally, facing towards the back of the upper jaw and are not moveable as are adder fangs. This makes it impossible for this snake to be held in the usual way. If gripped behind the head, it merely twists its head sideways to pierce a finger. It may also press the sharp tip of its tail against a person holding it, creating the impression that it is biting. To inject venom into its prey, it protrudes a fang, then moves its head over its prey while stabbing downwards.

Similar species

Often confused with a variety of other insignificant-looking snakes, including the purple-glossed snakes (*Amblyodipsas* sp.), the Natal Black Snake (*Macrelaps microlepidotus*) and the harmless Wolf Snake (*Lycophidion* sp.).

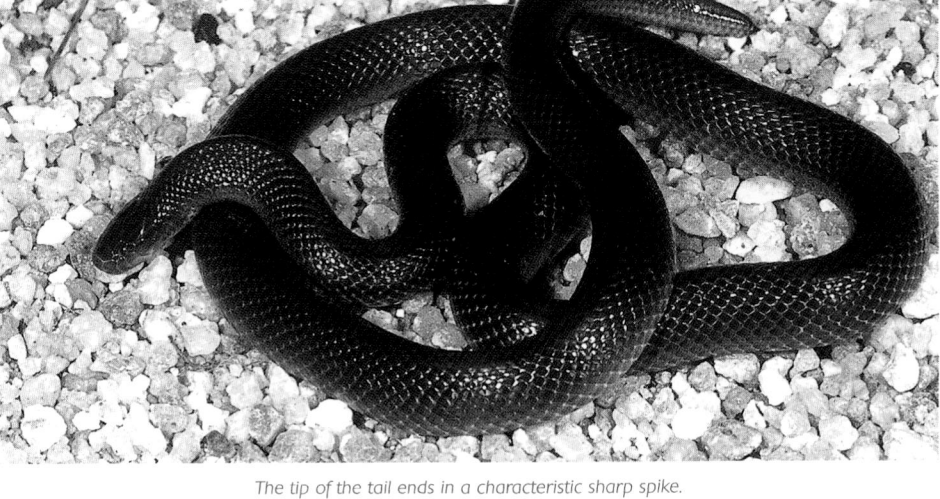

The tip of the tail ends in a characteristic sharp spike.

Enemies

Other snakes.

Food and feeding

Preys upon a variety of burrowing reptiles, frogs and small rodents, most of which are taken while in their burrows.

Reproduction

Oviparous, laying 3-7 eggs (27-36 x 10-12 mm) in mid-summer. The young measure 15 cm in length.

Danger to man

No fatalities have been recorded. However, this snake delivers an extremely painful bite that has led to the loss of fingers. Most victims are snake handlers. Bites are quite common in KwaZulu-Natal and Mpumalanga.

Venom

Bite victims experience intense local pain, swelling and often necrosis. Mild neurotoxic symptoms such as nausea and a dry throat may be present in the early stages. Antivenom is not effective against the venom of this snake and should therefore not be administered.

First-aid procedures

If you are certain of the snake's identity:
- Get the victim to a doctor or hospital where the bite must be treated symptomatically.
- Painkillers will be required.
- Otherwise resort to the first-aid measures discussed on page 9.

This snake cannot be held safely and you will, in all likelihood, get bitten if you hold one.

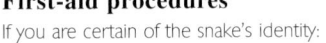

A similar-looking purple-glossed snake.

53

NATAL BLACK SNAKE

Macrelaps microlepidotus

Other names
Natalse Swartslang (A)

Average 60 cm
Maximum 1,2 m

LOOK OUT FOR
- A small head with reduced eyes.
- Usually uniform black to jet-black above.
- A docile snake that does not bite readily.

Preferred habitats
Damp localities in lowland forest and along streams in coastal bush.

Habits
Usually found beneath rotting logs or under stones, in leaf litter, animal burrows and in storm water drains. It may be seen moving about on warm overcast days, otherwise it surfaces on warm, damp nights. It is a docile snake that is very reluctant to bite.

Similar species
May be confused with the Stiletto Snake and the purple-glossed snakes.

Enemies
Other snakes.

Food and feeding
Feeds on frogs (especially rain frogs) legless lizards, snakes and small rodents. It grabs its prey and wraps a few coils around it and then chews to enable the venom to penetrate.

Reproduction
Oviparous, laying 3-10 eggs (38-56 × 23-31 mm) in summer. The young measure 20-29 cm in length.

Danger to man
The venom of this snake is not well studied, but is not thought to be fatal. Fortunately, the snake rarely bites.

This snake is often found beneath stones and rotting logs.

Venom
This snake does not often feature in snake-bite accidents but its bite may be serious. Loss of consciousness for up to 30 minutes has been recorded. Antivenom is not required as it has no effect in neutralising the venom of this snake.

First-aid procedures
- Immobilise and reassure the patient, who must lie down and be kept as quiet as possible.
- Apply a pressure bandage immediately (*see* page 9) and immobilise the limb with a splint to reduce the spread of venom.
- Loosen, but do not remove, the bandage if there is severe swelling.
- Transport promptly to hospital.

This burrowing snake seldom comes to the surface except on hot, damp nights and on hot overcast days.

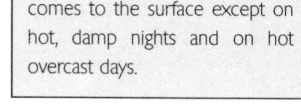

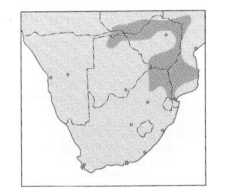

RUFOUS BEAKED SNAKE

Rhamphiophis rostratus

MILDLY VENOMOUS

Other names
Haakneusslang (A)

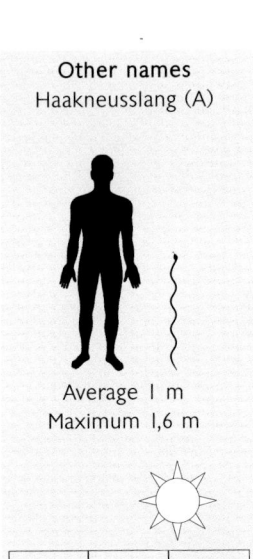

Average 1 m
Maximum 1,6 m

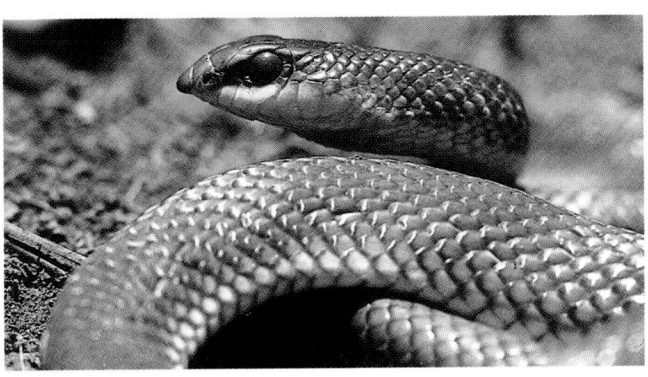

Note the dark stripe that extends through the eye of this snake.

LOOK OUT FOR.
- Conspicuous dark markings on either side of the head, from the nostril through the eye.
- A distinctive hooked 'beak'.

Preferred habitat
Bushveld or thorny sandveld areas in moist savanna.

Habits
A diurnal snake that spends much of its time in rodent burrows and termite mounds searching for food. It has the peculiar habit of jerking its elevated head from side to side. This snake may hiss but seldom attempts to bite.

Similar species
The female Boomslang and the Olive Grass Snake.

Enemies
Predatory birds and other snakes.

Food and feeding
Rodents, lizards, small snakes, frogs and small birds. Juveniles also feed on insects.

Reproduction
Oviparous, laying 7-18 eggs (34-42 × 22-24 mm) in mid-summer. The young measure 30 cm in length.

Danger to man
No danger to man.

Venom
Has virtually no effect on man.

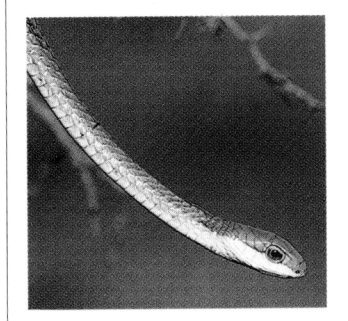

The similar female Boomslang lacks a dark stripe through the eye.

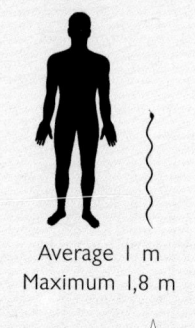

OLIVE GRASS SNAKE

Psammophis mossambicus

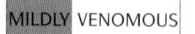

Other names
Olyfgrasslang (A)

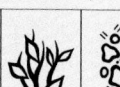

Average 1 m
Maximum 1,8 m

LOOK OUT FOR
- Nervous behaviour: dashes for the nearest cover when disturbed.
- Dark speckling on the upper lip.
- May lift up to a third of its body off the ground.

Preferred habitat
An inhabitant of moist savannna and lowland forest. Often found in the vicinity of water.

Habits
A robust, active and alert diurnal snake that dashes for cover when disturbed. It will remain hidden until flushed out. It lifts the front third of its body well off the ground like the Black Mamba. This snake has a very nervous disposition and retreats before one can approach closely.

Although mainly a ground-dwelling snake, the Olive Grass Snake may climb onto shrubs and bushes to bask. Many individuals have truncated tails: the result of injuries sustained during encounters with predators.

Did you know?
Snakes regularly survive for long periods, sometimes up to six months, without food. A large rat could take a week to digest and should sustain a snake for several weeks. Some of the less active snakes, like the Gaboon Adder, can survive comfortably on about one meal a month.

Similar species
The Black Mamba, the Rufous Beaked Snake and the Boomslang.

Enemies
Predatory birds and snakes.

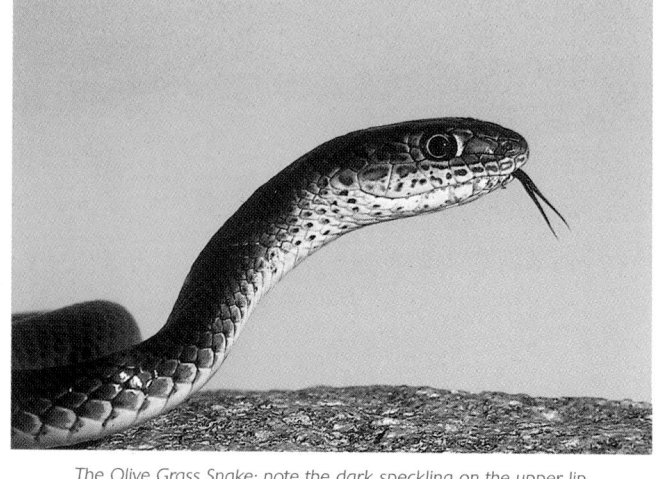

The Olive Grass Snake; note the dark speckling on the upper lip.

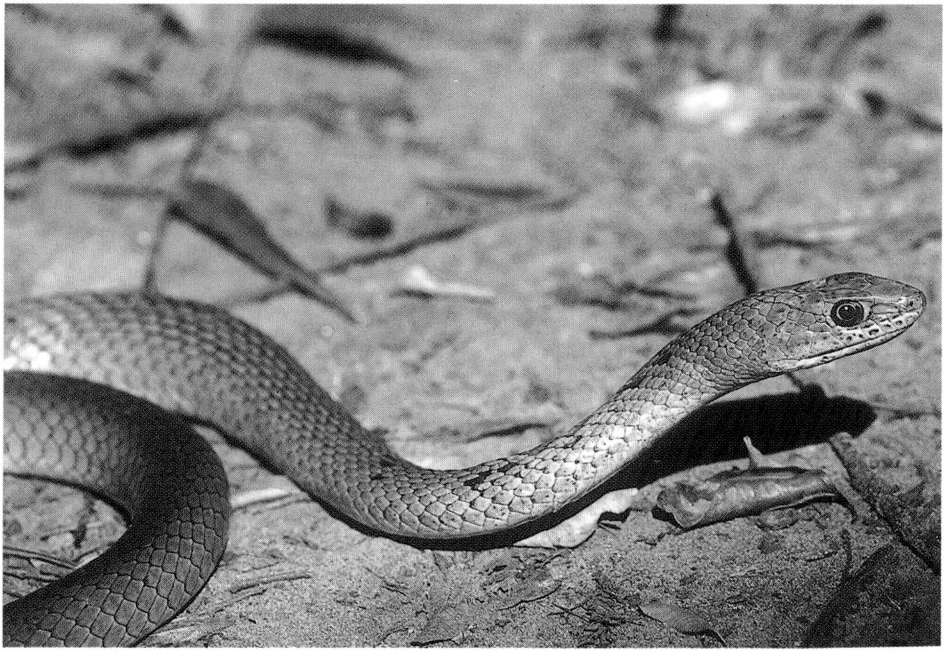

The Olive Grass Snake is essentially a ground-dweller.

Food and feeding

Feeds on lizards, small mammals, frogs and snakes, including the Black Mamba and the Puff Adder. Small birds are also taken.

Reproduction

Oviparous, laying 10-30 eggs (28-40 x 10-20 mm) in mid-summer. The young average 27-30 cm in length.

Did you know?
Snakes never lick their prey, nor do they cover their prey in saliva prior to swallowing it. A snake may, however, inspect its dead prey with its flickering tongue.

Danger to man

This snake is not considered to be of any danger to humans.

Venom

A mild venom that may cause local pain, swelling and occasionally nausea.

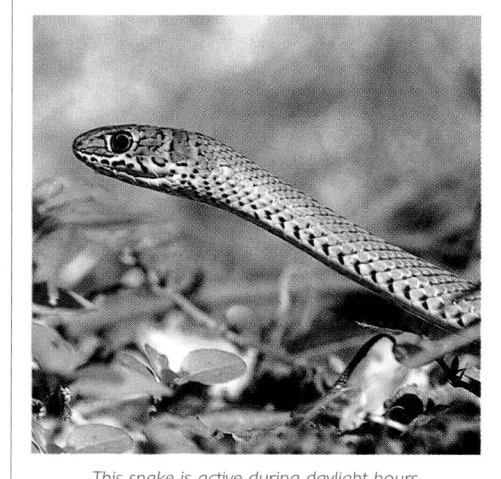

This snake is active during daylight hours.

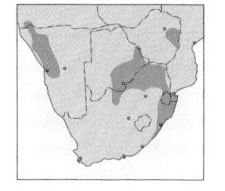

SHORT-SNOUTED GRASS SNAKE

Psammophis brevirostris

MILDLY VENOMOUS

Other names
Leopard Grass Snake (E)
Kortsnoetgrasslang (A)

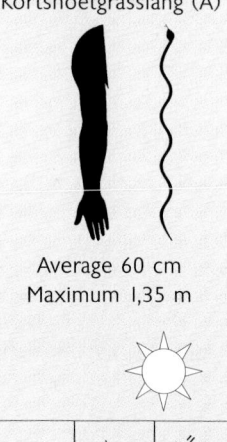

Average 60 cm
Maximum 1,35 m

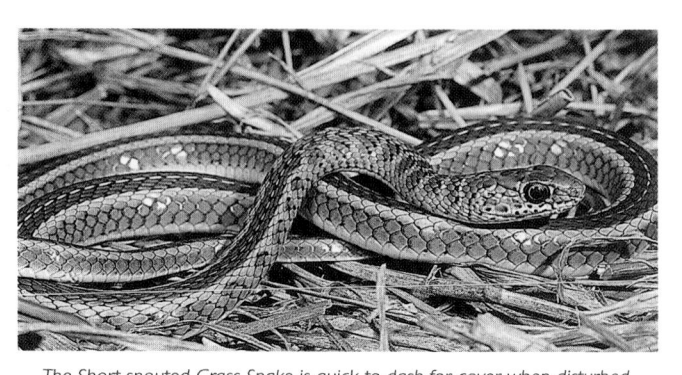

The Short-snouted Grass Snake is quick to dash for cover when disturbed.

LOOK OUT FOR
- Stripes along the body.
- Dashes for the closest cover when disturbed.
- Active during the day.

Preferred habitat
Grassland, moist savanna and lowland forest in the east, and Karoo and Namib Desert in the west.

Habits
An alert, fast-moving snake (often seen crossing roads), usually disappearing before it is properly identified. It is quick to dash for cover when disturbed and will remain motionless until flushed out. Although primarily a ground-dweller, it often ventures into low shrubs to bask.

Similar species
Resembles sand and grass snakes and may be mistaken for a small Black Mamba or a female Boomslang.

Enemies
Birds of prey and other snakes.

Food and feeding
Snakes, lizards, rodents and small birds.

Reproduction
Oviparous, laying 4-15 eggs (23-40 × 10-20 mm) in summer. The young measure 19-27 cm in length.

Danger to man
No danger to man.

Venom
Not thought to have any harmful effect on humans.

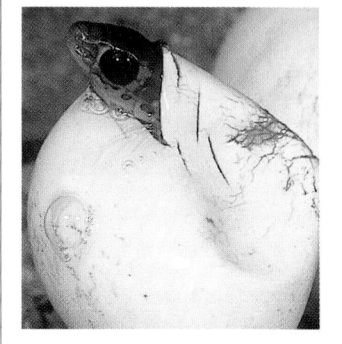

A hatchling cuts through the egg.

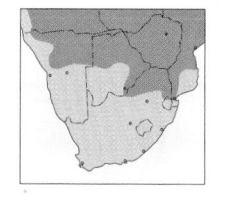

STRIPE-BELLIED SAND SNAKE *Psammophis subtaeniatus*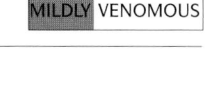

Other names
Gestreepte Sandslang, Geelpenssandslang (A)

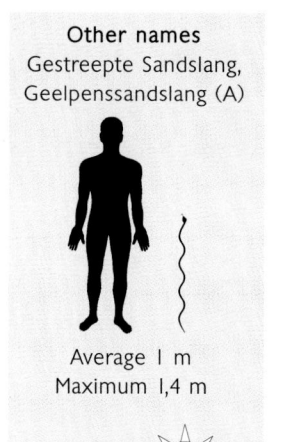

Average 1 m
Maximum 1,4 m

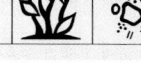

LOOK OUT FOR
- Stripes along its body.
- A lemon-yellow belly.
- Moves off very quickly and freezes when it gets into the closest shrub.
- Frequents water.
- Active during the day.

Preferred habitat
Both arid and moist savanna.

Habits
This is probably southern Africa's fastest snake. It is common throughout most of its range, especially in the drier regions. Like many of the other sand snakes, it is active during the day, often during the hottest hours. The Stripe-bellied Sand Snake is often found near water.

This snake moves off rapidly when disturbed, only to freeze when it gets into the nearest bush or shrub. There it relies on its excellent camouflage to escape detection. Though a ground-dweller, it ventures into shrubs and low bushes either to bask or to seek out food.

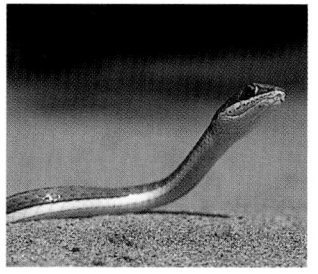

This is probably southern Africa's fastest snake.

Similar species
Easily confused with the other sand snakes and the equally harmless Striped Skaapsteker.

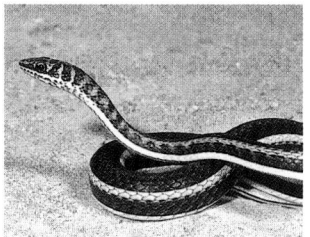

Specimen from the Pilanesberg area.

Enemies
Predatory birds and other snakes.

Food and feeding
Prefers lizards but also eats frogs, rodents and small birds.

Reproduction
Oviparous, laying 4-10 eggs in summer (32 × 12 mm). The young are about 20 cm in length.

Danger to man
No danger to man.

Venom
Not thought to have any harmful effect on humans.

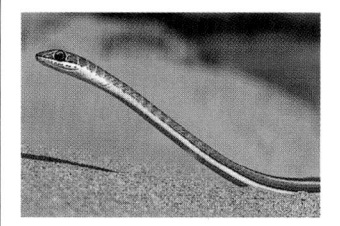

The lemon-yellow belly is diagnostic.

59

SPOTTED SKAAPSTEKER

Psammophylax rhombeatus

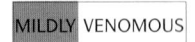 MILDLY VENOMOUS

Other names
Rhombic Skaapsteker (E);
Gevlekte Skaapsteker (A)

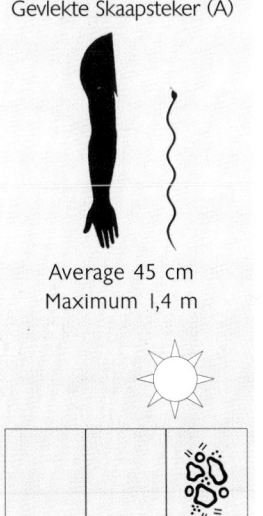

Average 45 cm
Maximum 1,4 m

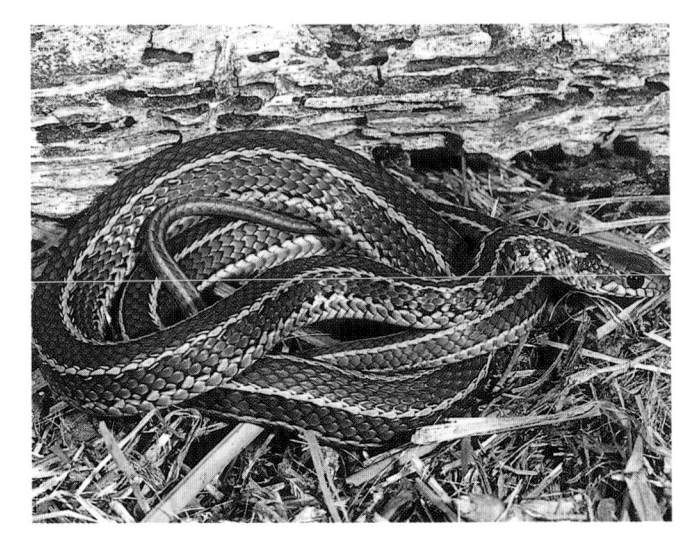

A Spotted Skaapsteker from the KwaZulu-Natal Drakensberg.

LOOK OUT FOR
- Dashes for cover where it is well camouflaged.
- Nervous and quick moving.
- Active during the day.

Preferred habitats
Found from the coast to mountain tops where it inhabits fynbos, grassland and moist savanna.

Habits
A diurnal snake that actively hunts its prey. It is nervous and quick-moving, disappearing into grass when disturbed. There it freezes and will usually coil around a tuft of grass. It is well camouflaged and difficult to find.

Similar species
May be confused with some of the equally harmless sand and grass snakes.

Enemies
Predatory birds and other snakes.

Food and feeding
Mostly feeds on rodents, lizards, birds and frogs.

Did you know?
Snakes often change colour gradually from the juvenile to the adult stage. Juvenile snakes tend to be brighter in colour than the adults. Prior to shedding, snakes often become dull in colour as the old skin is damaged, but are a lot more attractive immediately after shedding. Colour changes occur over a long period and are clearly noticeable only after many old skins have been shed.

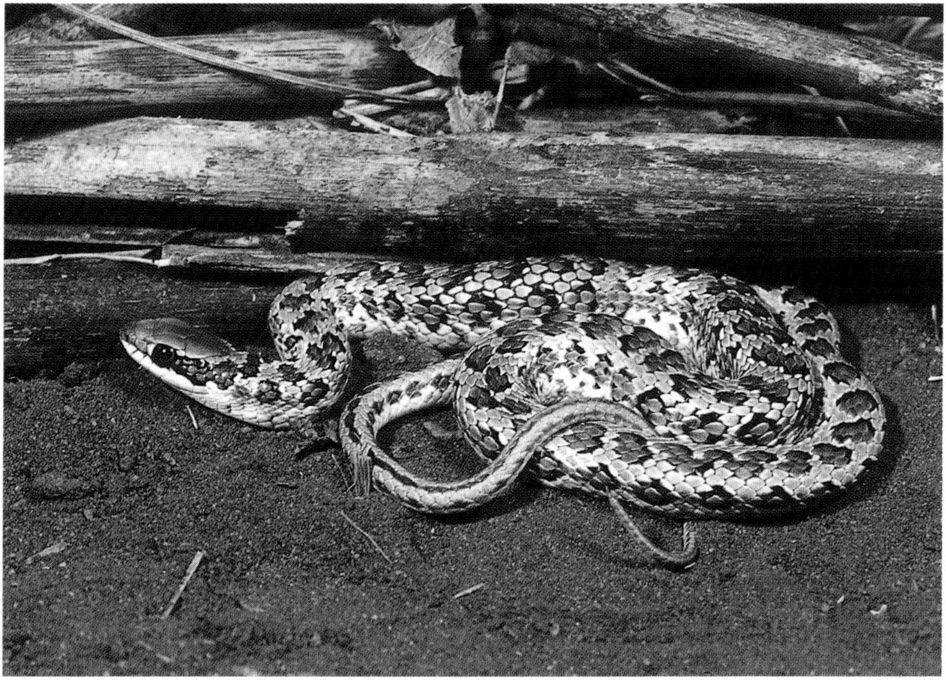

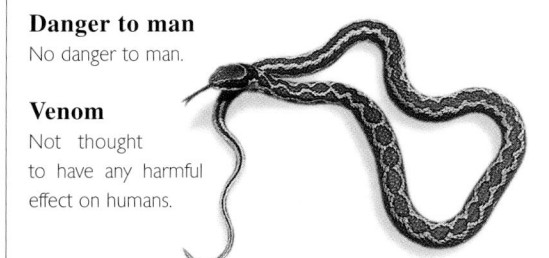

A Spotted Skaapsteker from the Western Cape.

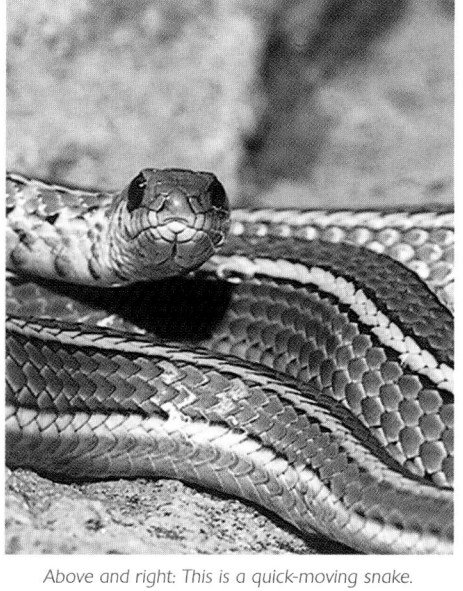

Above and right: This is a quick-moving snake.

Reproduction
Oviparous, laying 8-30 eggs (20-35 × 12-18 mm) in summer. Females have been found coiled around their eggs. The young measure 16-24 cm.

Danger to man
No danger to man.

Venom
Not thought to have any harmful effect on humans.

> **What's in a name?**
> The common name 'Skaapsteker' (Afrikaans for sheep stabber) is misleading as this snake is not capable of killing sheep.

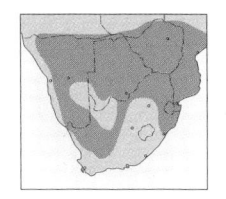

TIGER SNAKE

Telescopus species

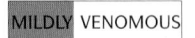
MILDLY VENOMOUS

Other names

Tierslang (A)

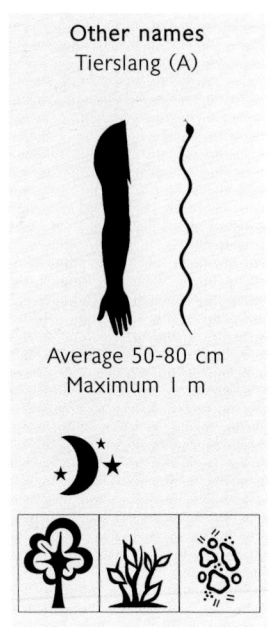

Average 50-80 cm
Maximum 1 m

Preferred habitat

Rocky regions in the Namib Desert, Karoo, arid and moist savanna and lowland forest where it shelters under bark, loose flakes of rock and in rock crevices.

Did you know?

Smaller snakes live for only a year or two, but large pythons may live up to 25 years or even more. The average cobra or mamba probably lives for about five to ten years.

Habits

A nocturnal snake that spends most of the day concealed in rock crevices or under the bark of trees. Though largely a ground-dweller, it does venture into trees, shrubs and old buildings, where it hunts for food. During summer, after rains, Tiger Snakes often cross tarred roads and as a result many individuals are killed by passing vehicles.

Like the Red-lipped Herald Snake, this snake puts on an impressive display when threatened or cornered, raising its head off the ground and striking viciously.

LOOK OUT FOR

- Has 22-59 dark brown or black crossbars or blotches on the body and tail.
- May lift its head and strike out viciously if threatened.
- Often found on tarred roads after heavy rains.
- Active at night.

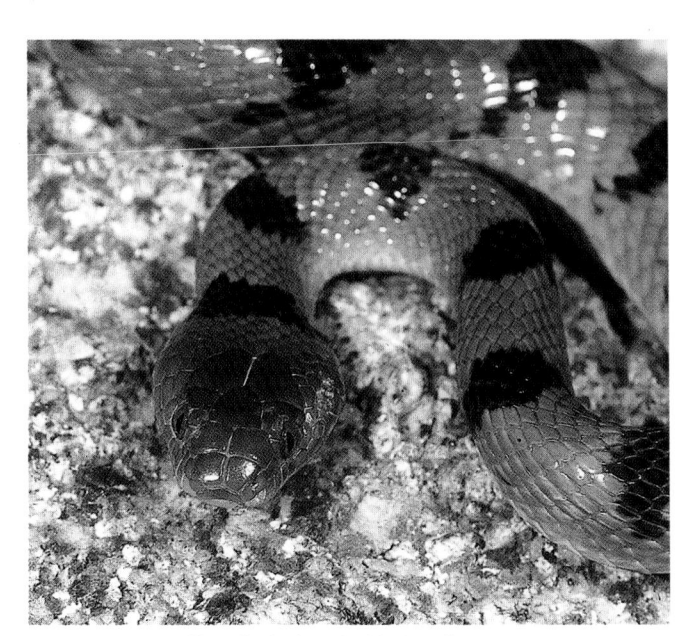

Tiger Snake from the Northern Province.

62

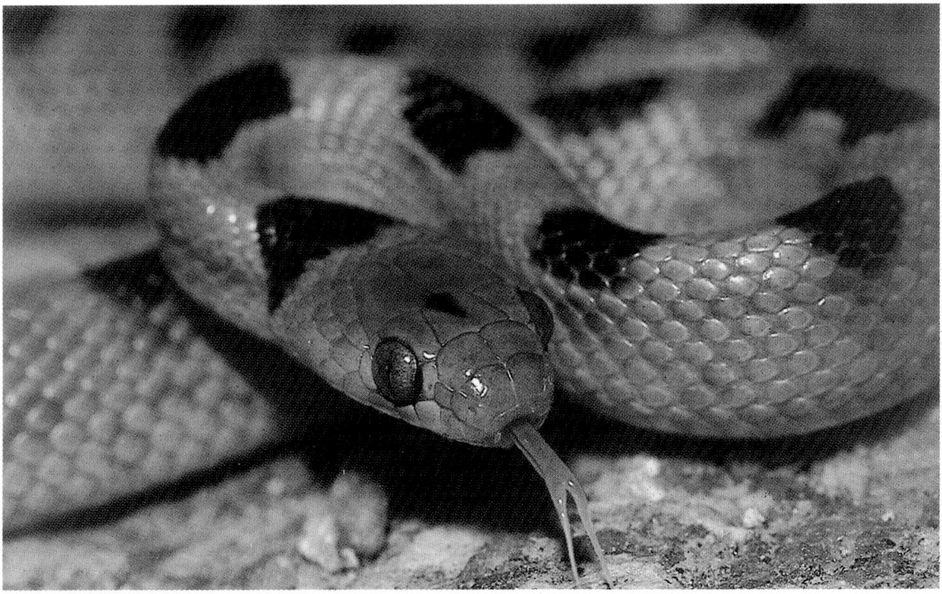

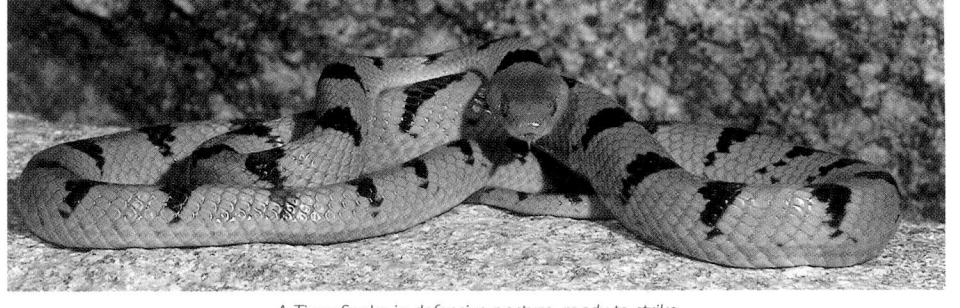

A Tiger Snake flickering its tongue. Note the vertical pupil of this nocturnal snake.

Similar species

May be confused with the Coral Snake and also the Western Barred Spitting Cobra.

Enemies

Other snakes.

Food and feeding

Mainly lizards, especially geckos. Fledgling birds, bats and small rodents are also taken.

Reproduction

Oviparous, laying from 3-20 eggs (10-17 x 24-55 mm) during the summer. The hatchlings measure from 17-23 cm in length.

Danger to man

No danger to man.

Venom

Not thought to have any harmful effect on man.

A Tiger Snake in defensive posture, ready to strike.

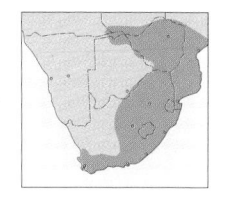

HERALD SNAKE

Crotaphopeltis hotamboeia

MILDLY VENOMOUS

Other names
Red-lipped Snake (E);
Rooilipslang (A)

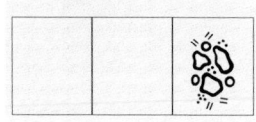

Average 45 cm
Maximum I m

Preferred habitat
Very common in marshy areas in fynbos, moist savanna and lowland forest.

Habits
Common and widespread, it is often found in gardens where it seeks shelter in rockeries, under building rubble and in compost heaps. Because of its nocturnal habits, people often incorrectly refer to it as a Night Adder.

It preys predominantly on toads and prefers damp localities. When threatened, the Herald Snake will raise its flattened head horizontally, while hissing and striking with its mouth agape. It bites readily. This and

the Brown House Snake are without doubt the two most common garden snakes in southern Africa.

Did you know?
Contrary to popular belief, snakes are not wet and slimy. In fact they are perfectly dry. A snake may well be wet after a swim or as a result of slithering through wet vegetation, but it is never slimy. Some snakes, because of their shiny, highly reflective skins, may appear to be wet, but they are in fact dry.

LOOK OUT FOR
• Often bright red to orange markings on the upper lip.
• Head is usually much darker than the body, which may have scattered, lighter flecks.
• Found in damp places.
• When threatened may flatten its head horizontally and strike with intent, as would an adder.
• Active at night.

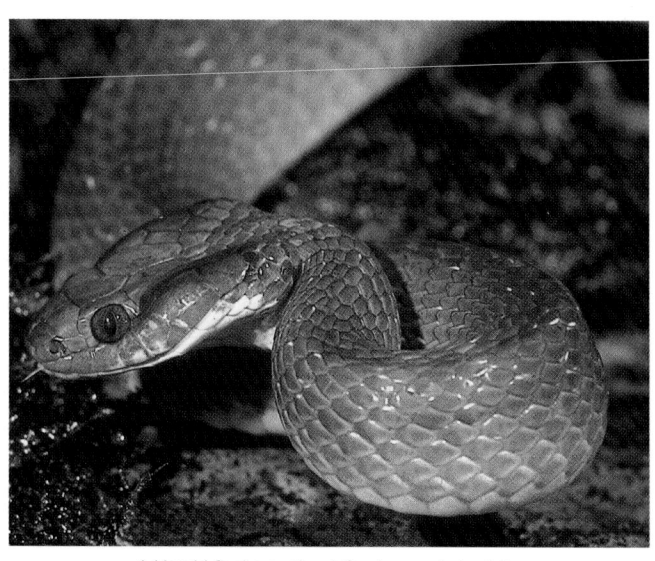

A Herald Snake on the defensive, ready to strike.

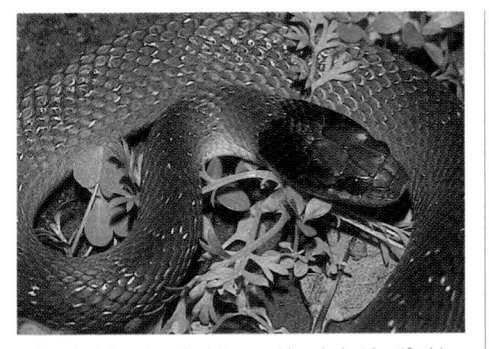

The dark head and white speckling help identify this snake in most instances.

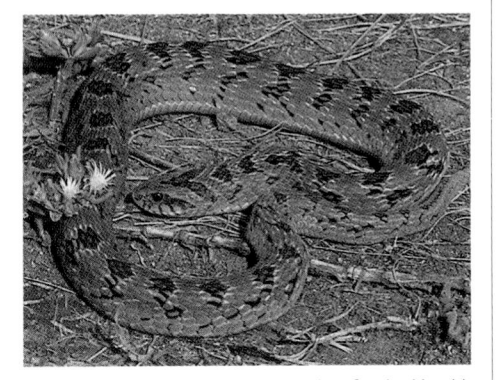

The Night Adder is commonly mistaken for the Herald Snake despite the fact that the two are dissimilar.

Similar species

Even though there is no resemblance, this snake is often incorrectly identified as a Night Adder.

Enemies

Other snakes.

Food and feeding

Feeds largely on frogs and toads, including the rain frog. Once this snake grabs a toad in its jaws, it hangs onto it while its mild venom takes effect.

Reproduction

Oviparous, laying 6-19 eggs (25-32 x 10-13 mm) in early summer. The young measure 8-18 cm in length.

Danger to man

No danger to man.

Venom

Not thought to have any harmful effect on man.

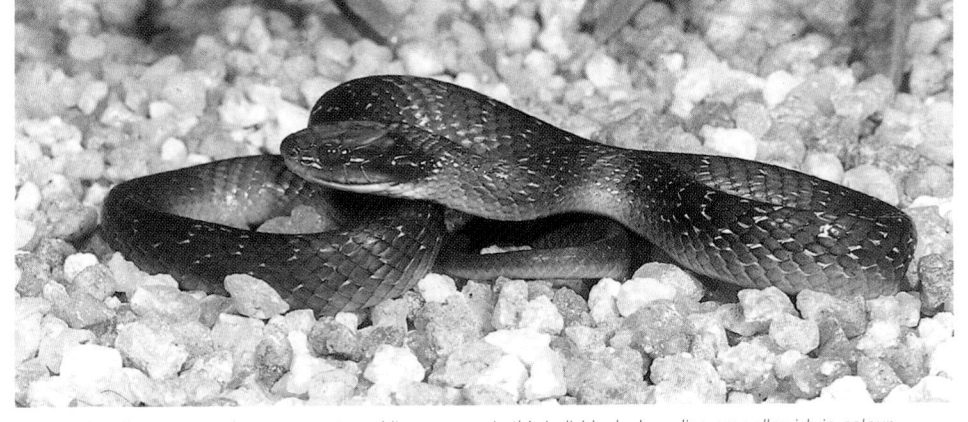

Not all specimens show orange to red lips, as seen in this individual whose lips are yellowish in colour.

CAPE CENTIPEDE-EATER

Aparallactus capensis

MILDLY VENOMOUS

Other names

Black-headed Snake (E)
Kaapse Honderd-
pootvreter; Swart-
kopslang (A)

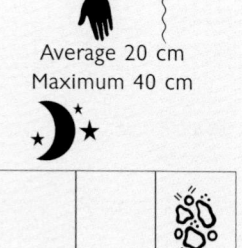

Average 20 cm
Maximum 40 cm

Preferred habitat

Commonly found in old termite mounds in lowland forest, moist savanna and grassland.

Habits

This slender snake is common throughout its range and is usually found in disused termite mounds and under logs and stones. It is nocturnal and is very active after rains. Many individuals may inhabit a single termite mound to which they are attracted by warmth, suitable shelter and food. The Centipede-eater bites readily when handled but its teeth are minute and seldom pierce skin. It is often caught by inexperienced snake collectors but does not do well in captivity and soon starves to death.

Similar species

This snake has very distinct, dark markings on the head and neck and cannot easily be confused with other snake species.

Enemies

Other snakes, spiders and scorpions.

Food and feeding

Feeds on centipedes, which it seizes and then chews up and down the length of the body until its venom takes effect. If the centipede bites the snake, it will release its prey and start the chewing process all over again. The centipede is swallowed head first. Occassionally centipedes may kill the snake during the attack and then proceed to eat the predator.

LOOK OUT FOR

- A small slender snake.
- Brownish in colour with black markings on the head and neck.
- Often found in deserted termite mounds.
- Active at night, especially after rains.

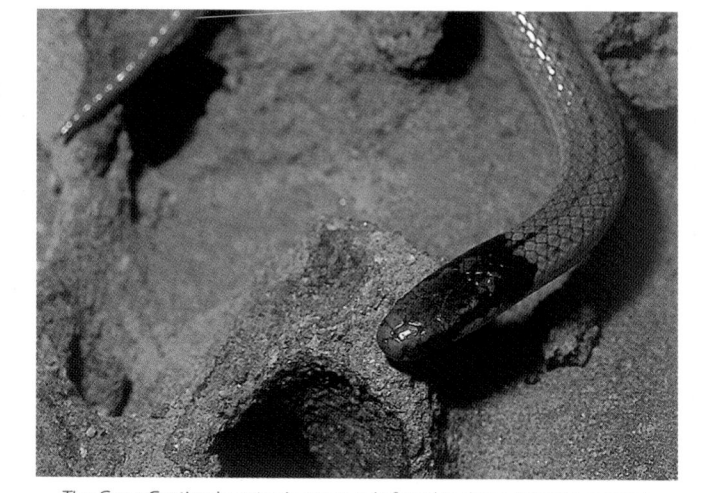

The Cape Centipede-eater is commonly found in disused termite mounds.

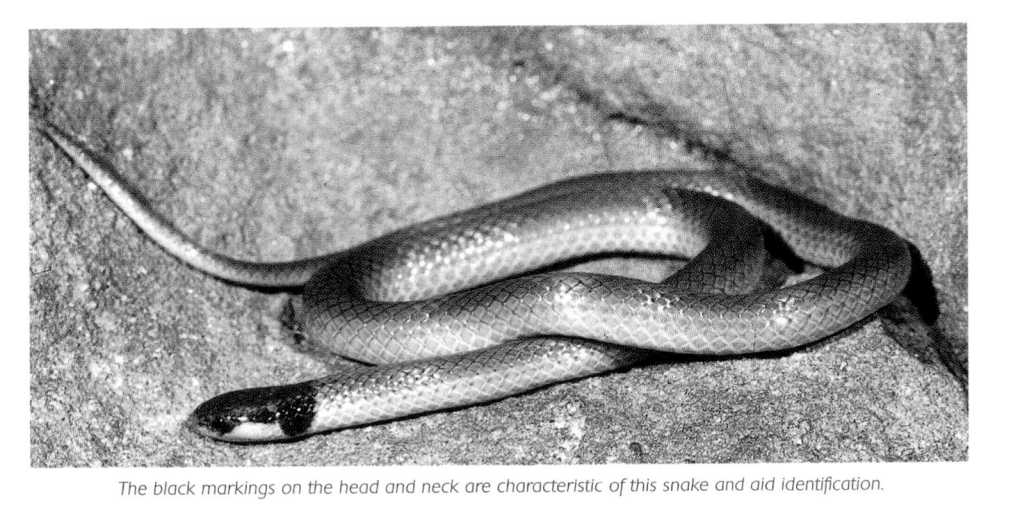

The black markings on the head and neck are characteristic of this snake and aid identification.

Reproduction

Oviparous, laying 2-4 elongate eggs (32 × 4-5 mm) during the summer. The young measure from 9-12 cm in length and are perfect replicas of the adults, complete with the dark head.

Danger to man

No danger to man.

Venom

Not thought to have any effect on man.

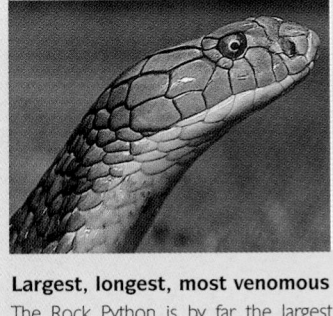

Largest, longest, most venomous
The Rock Python is by far the largest snake in southern Africa, while the Black Mamba is the largest *venomous* snake in our region. However, the longest snake in the world – exceeding eight metres in length – is the Reticulated Python of Asia. The Anaconda of South America is by far the *bulkiest* snake, while the King Cobra of Asia is the largest *venomous* snake in the world.

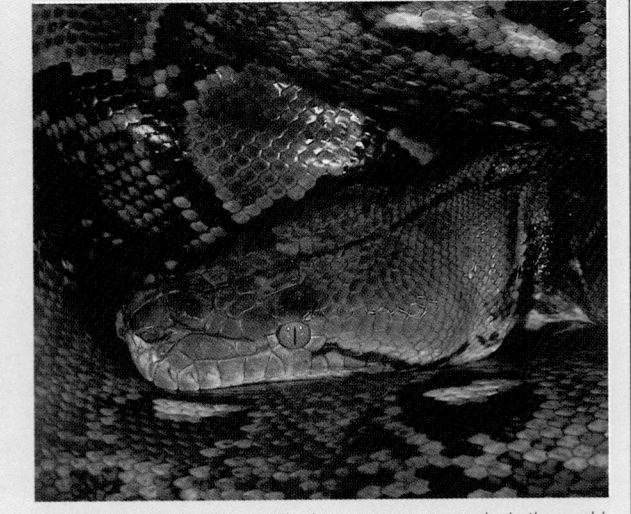

Top left: Asia's King Cobra is the largest venomous snake in the world. Above: The Reticulated Python, also from Asia, is the world's longest snake, growing in excess of eight metres.

SOUTHERN AFRICAN ROCK PYTHON

Python sebae

Other names
Suider Afrikaanse
Luislang (A)

Average 3-4 m
Maximum 6,5 m

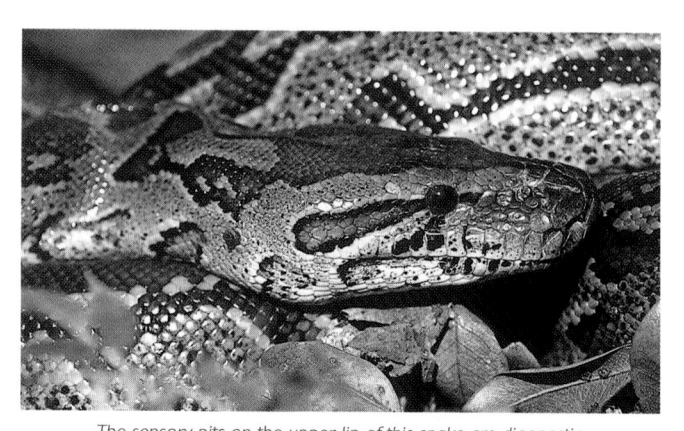

The sensory pits on the upper lip of this snake are diagnostic.

LOOK OUT FOR
- A large, bulky snake.
- Several heat sensory pits on the upper lip.
- Likes to bask in the sun, especially after a large meal.
- Partial to water and often dives into deep pools where it can remain submerged for long periods of time.
- Most active at night.

Preferred habitat
Fairly widespread, preferring rocky outcrops in arid and moist savanna as well as in lowland forest.

Habits
Most active at night, though very fond of basking – especially after a large meal. It ambushes its prey, latches on with its powerful recurved teeth and constricts it. Despite popular belief, it does not crush its prey to death and never breaks any bones in the process. It is also incorrect that a python has to anchor its tail onto a tree before it can constrict its prey.

Pythons are extremely valuable as they control rodent populations, especially dassies and cane rats. Unfortunately, they have been killed indiscriminately in the past and this persists today. The Southern African Rock Python is listed as vulnerable in the latest *South African Red Data Book – Reptiles and Amphibians* and may not be killed or captured. Both its skin and fat are still used in traditional medicine.

Did you know?
Some snakes, including pythons, boas and American rattlesnakes, have heat sensory pits which enable them to detect minute differences in temperature and accurately locate warm-blooded prey in pitch darkness. Rattlesnakes and Pit Vipers have two heat sensory pits – one on either side of the head between the eye and the nostril. Pythons and boas, however, have a series of heat sensory pits situated along the upper lip.

68

Similar species

This large, bulky snake cannot easily be confused with other snakes.

Enemies

Mongooses, meerkats, crocodiles, wild dogs, hyaenas, honey badgers and other snakes. Many are killed while crossing roads. Some are also killed for their skin and fat.

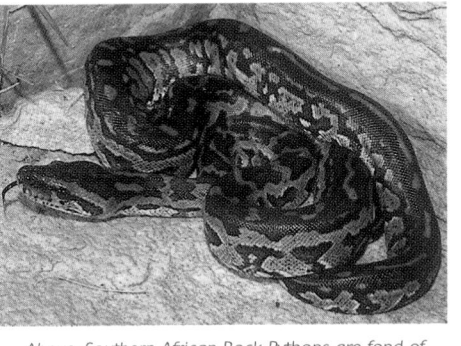

Above: Southern African Rock Pythons are fond of basking, especially after a large meal.
Top: A juvenile Southern African Rock Python.

Food and feeding

Diet includes dassies, cane rats, hares, monkeys, small antelope and game birds. Fish, monitor lizards or leguaans, and crocodiles are also taken. Juveniles feed largely on ground-living birds and rodents.

Reproduction

Oviparous, laying 30-50 eggs (in exceptional cases more than 100) depending on the size of the female.

The eggs are about 10 cm in diameter (a bit smaller than a tennis ball) and weigh 130-160 grams. Once the female has deposited her eggs in a suitable site, such as a hollowed-out termite mound or ant-bear hole, it will coil around her eggs and remain there until they hatch. During this period she will not feed but may leave the eggs to drink. The eggs hatch after two to three months and the young, measuring 45-60 cm in length, move off on their own, unprotected by the female.

Danger to man

Pythons have been known to kill people in the past but today large individuals are very rare. Because of the python's size and the fact that it has numerous strong, recurved teeth, a bite may cause a fair amount of tissue damage and the victim may even need stitches.

First-aid procedures

■ A bite from a python must be treated as a dirty wound: washed and disinfected and watched for signs of sepsis. Medical advice should be sought.

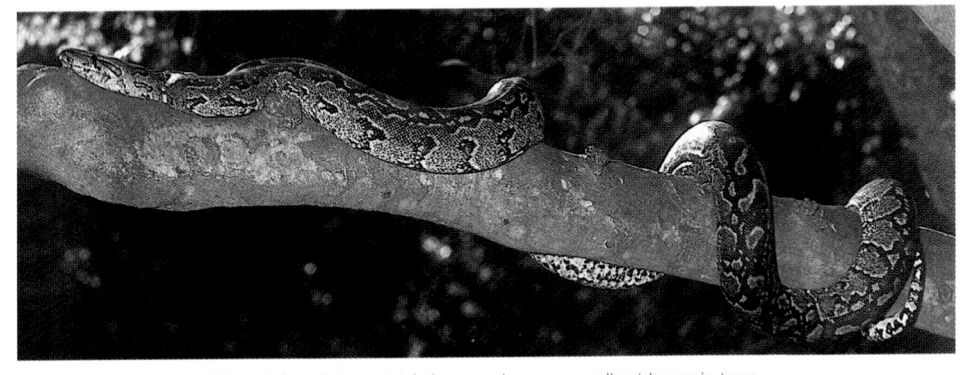

Though largely terrestrial, these snakes are equally at home in trees.

69

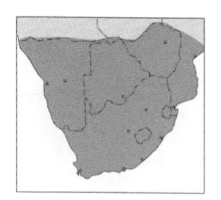

BROWN HOUSE SNAKE

Lamprophis fuliginosus

HARMLESS

Other names
Bruin Huisslang (A)

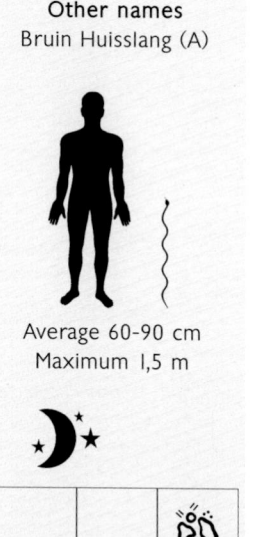

Average 60-90 cm
Maximum 1,5 m

Preferred habitat
Found just about everywhere; common around human dwellings, hence the common name.

Habits
A common nocturnal constrictor that forages for rodents. It is often found around houses but, because of its

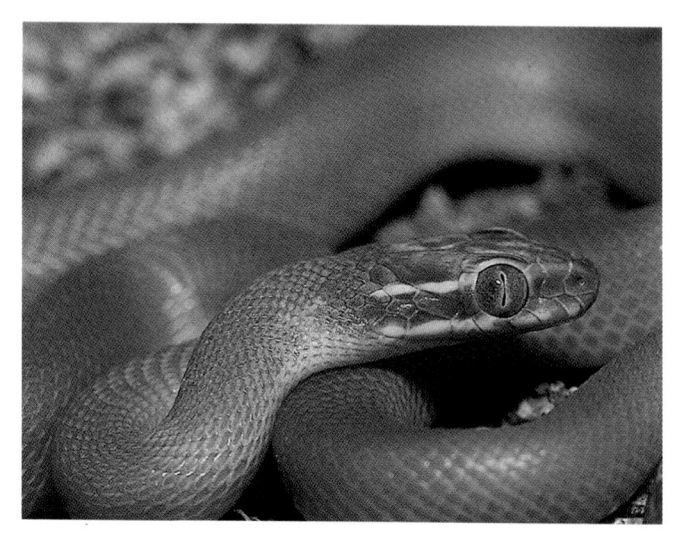

The two light stripes on either side of the head are characteristic of this snake and will help in identification.

LOOK OUT FOR
• Usually has two light stripes on either side of the head: one from the nose through the eye to the back of the head and the other from the eye to the angle of the jaw.
• Common around human dwellings.
• Active at night.

Did you know?
Many snakes, such as the Brown House Snake and the Spotted Bush Snake have adapted well to urbanisation and seek shelter in compost heaps, under building rubble and in rockeries where they feel secure and have access to a source of food such as rodents, toads and lizards.

nocturnal habits, is not seen that often except during cleaning-up operations when it may be found beneath building rubble, in compost heaps or even in tool sheds and outbuildings.

It preys largely on rodents, securing its prey with its sharp teeth and then constricting it. This snake has the ability to devour an entire rodent family in one session. The Brown House Snake may bite readily if threatened.

70

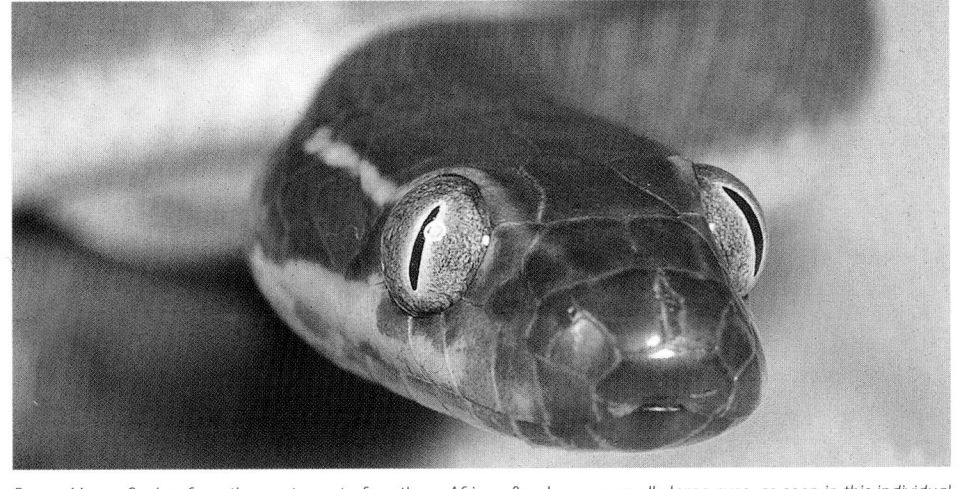

Brown House Snakes from the west coast of southern Africa often have unusually large eyes, as seen in this individual.

Similar species

Large individuals resemble small pythons.

Enemies

Several snakes, including the File Snake, cobras and sand snakes. It is also preyed upon by birds of prey, particularly owls. It is often killed by humans when encountered in residential gardens.

Food and feeding

Mainly rodents and other small vertebrates including bats. Lizards, especially skinks, are also taken.

Reproduction

Oviparous, laying 8-18 eggs (30 × 15 mm) in summer. The young measure 19-26 cm in length.

Danger to man

None.

> **Did you know?**
> Large snakes never stop growing, but just grow less and less as they get older.

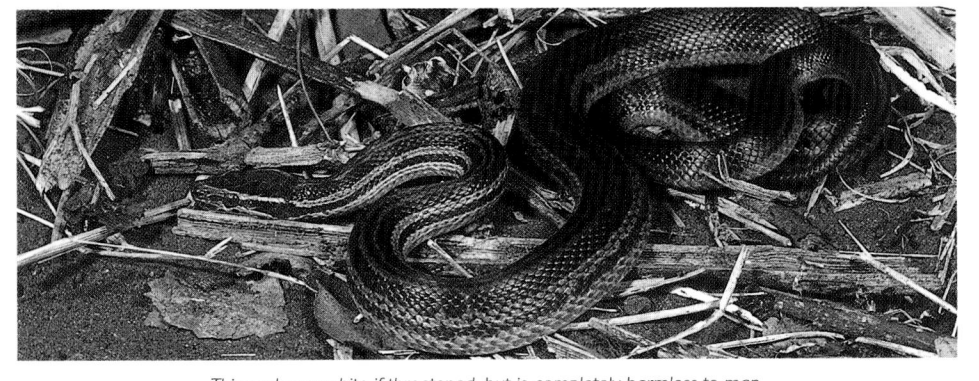

This snake may bite if threatened, but is completely harmless to man.

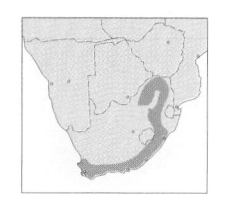

OLIVE HOUSE SNAKE

Lamprophis inornatus

HARMLESS

Other names
Black House Snake (E)
Nagslang;
Olyfhuisslang (A)

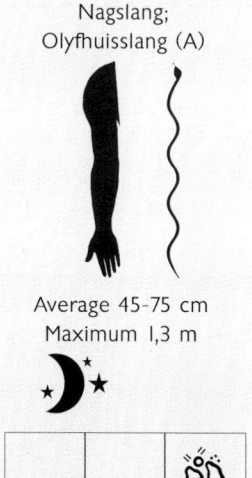

Average 45-75 cm
Maximum 1,3 m

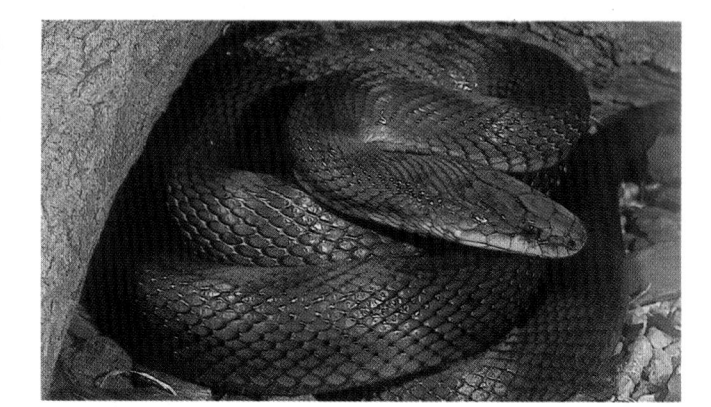

The harmless Olive House Snake (above) could be mistaken for several uniformly coloured snakes, including the Black Mamba.

LOOK OUT FOR
- Python-like in appearance, but not in colour.
- Strictly terrestrial, seldom venturing into trees or bushes.
- Active at night.

Did you know?
Most snakes swim well, with the exception of some of the burrowing species. Even sluggish land-dwellers like the Puff Adder swim easily across dams and rivers. Some, such as the python, like to dive deep into pools where they can remain submerged for long periods of time.

Preferred habitat
Moist savanna, lowland forest and fynbos, where it favours.

Habits
Very similar in habits to the Brown House Snake but prefers moister habitats. This snake is not nearly as common as the Brown House Snake.

It is partial to rubble and debris, and is also found near human dwellings.

Similar species
Could be mistaken for a variety of other uniformly coloured snakes, including the Black Mamba.

Enemies
Predatory birds and other snakes.

Food and feeding
This snake feeds on lizards, rodents and snakes.

Reproduction
Oviparous, laying 5-15 eggs (32-45 × 20-25 mm) in summer. The young measure 19-24 cm in length.

Danger to man
None.

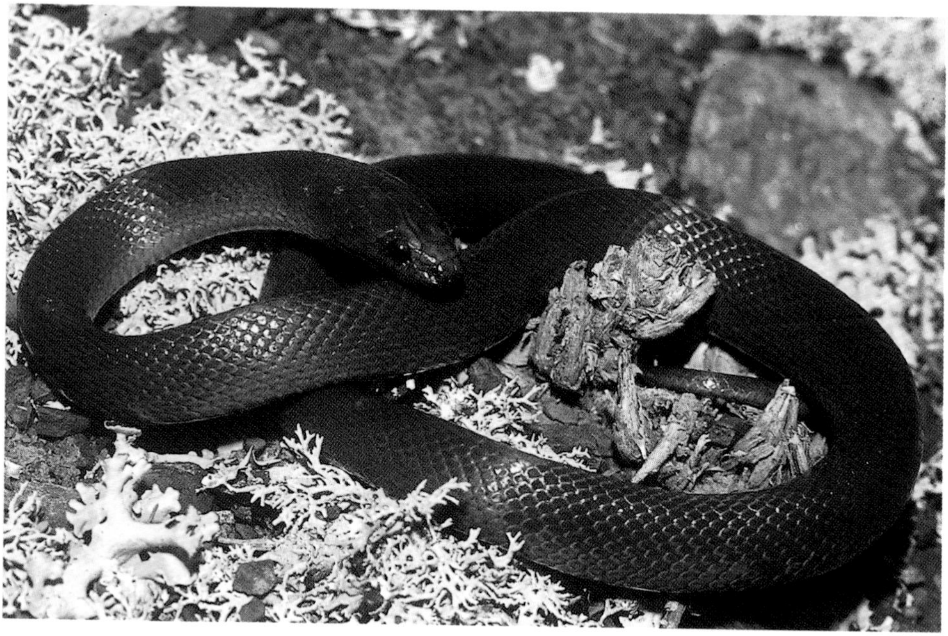

This snake is strictly terrestrial and seldom ventures into trees or bushes.

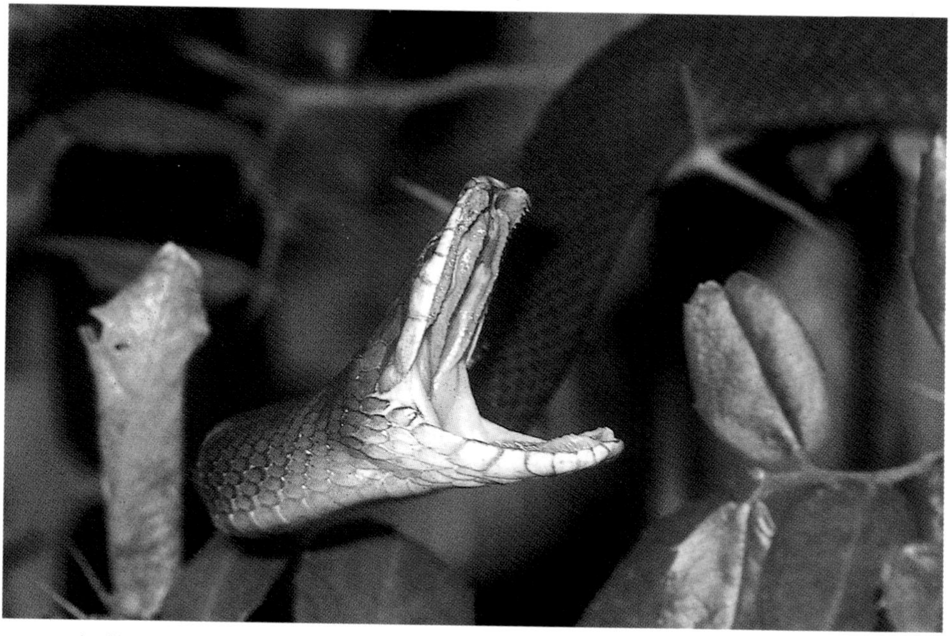

An Olive House Snake yawning; note the small teeth. This snake has no fangs and is not venomous.

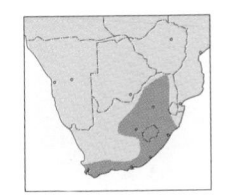

AURORA HOUSE SNAKE

Lamprophis aurora

HARMLESS

Other names
Auroraslang (A)

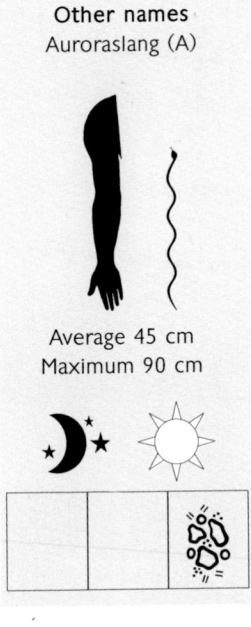

Average 45 cm
Maximum 90 cm

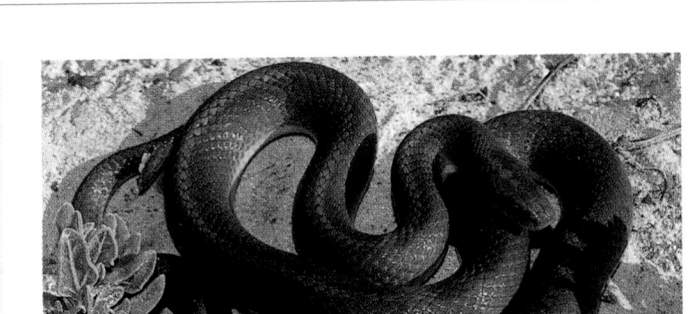

The distinct orange line down the back of this snake makes it easy to identify.

LOOK OUT FOR
- Uniform olive-green above with a distinct yellow to orange stripe down the back.
- Strictly terrestrial, seldom venturing into trees or bushes.
- Nocturnal, but may bask in the early morning or late afternoon.
- Often active on overcast days.

Preferred habitat
Favours damp localities in grasslands, moist savanna, lowland forest and also fynbos.

Habits
A colourful, nocturnal snake that may bask in the early mornings or late afternoons. It may also emerge on overcast days. The Aurora House Snake is very secretive and is seldom seen. It is a harmless constrictor and seldom attempts to bite.

Similar species
Juveniles may be confused with the striped phase of the Harlequin Snake (*Homoroselaps lacteus*).

Enemies
Snakes and predatory birds. Habitat destruction around Johannesburg has had an effect on local populations.

Food and feeding
Nestling rodents, lizards and frogs.

Reproduction
Oviparous, laying 8-12 eggs (35-44 × 19-20 mm) in summer. The young measure 20 cm in length.

Danger to man
None.

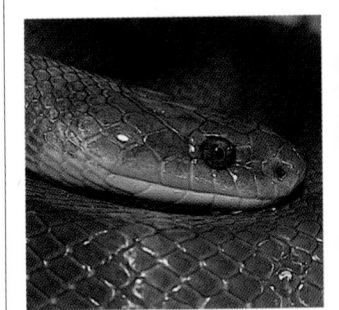

Aurora House Snake

74

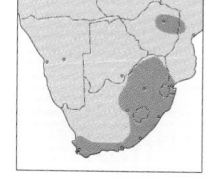

COMMON BROWN WATER SNAKE

Lycodonomorphus rufulus

Other names
Bruin Waterslang (A)

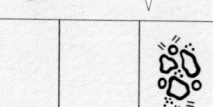

Average 45 cm
Maximum 85 cm

LOOK OUT FOR
- Plain dark blackish brown above, with a beautiful mother-of-pearl underside.
- Excellent swimmer.
- Largely active at night.

Preferred habitat
The wetter eastern half of southern Africa. Prefers rivers, streams, vleis and dams in grasslands, moist savanna, lowland forest and fynbos.

Habits
A nocturnal, aquatic snake that swims very well. Usually confined to very damp localities near streams and rivers. Although it is mainly active at night, it often hunts along shaded streams during the day.

This snake is common throughout much of its range and can be found beneath rocks, logs and other debris. Zulu people believe it to be very dangerous and call it *ivuzamanzi*. It is, in fact, a shy harmless snake.

This snake is usually confined to damp localities.

Enemies
Monitor lizards or leguaans, predatory birds and snakes.

Similar species
May be confused with other harmless snakes such as the Brown House Snake. Distinguished by its plain colour.

Food and feeding
A powerful constrictor that feeds on frogs, tadpoles, small fish and occasionally nestlings and rodents.

Reproduction
Oviparous, laying 6-23 eggs (12-21 × 20-24 mm) in mid-summer. The young measure 15-22 cm in length.

Danger to man
None.

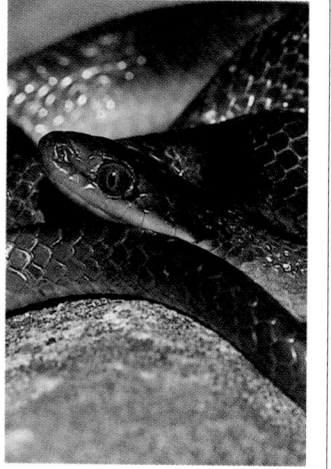

Common Brown Water Snake

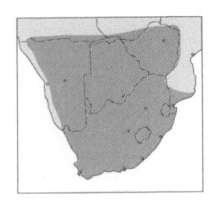

MOLE SNAKE

Pseudaspis cana

Other names
Molslang (A)

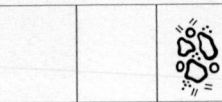

Average 1-1,4 m
Maximum 2 m

Preferred habitat
A variety of habitats including mountainous regions and even desert. Particularly common in sandy scrub-covered and grassveld regions.

Habits
A large powerful constrictor with a pointed snout and a small head very well adapted for its burrowing existence. It spends most of its time underground in search of food. Here it pushes its way through soft sand in search of moles and other rodents. Its prey is usually seized by the head and constricted.

Adult males are known to engage in combat during the mating season, biting one another and inflicting nasty wounds, which often result in permanent scars. The Mole Snake, although not venomous, can be quite vicious when threatened and will hiss and lunge forward with its mouth agape. Unfortunately, this useful snake is often mistaken for a cobra or mamba and is usually killed on sight.

Similar species
May be confused with the Black Mamba or a cobra, especially the Cape Cobra.

LOOK OUT FOR
- Varies tremendously in colour from nearly black to light brown. Juveniles often have rhombic markings.
- Pointed snout and small head.
- Spends much of its time underground in animal burrows.

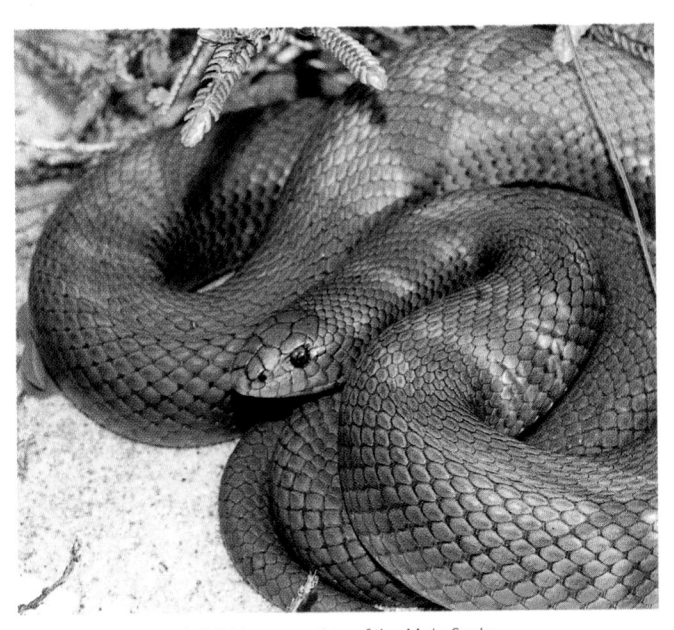

A light brown variety of the Mole Snake.

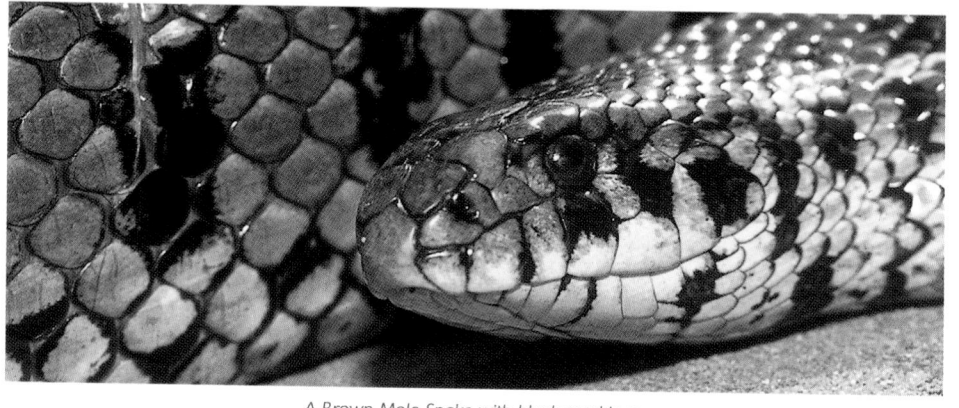

A Brown Mole Snake with black markings.

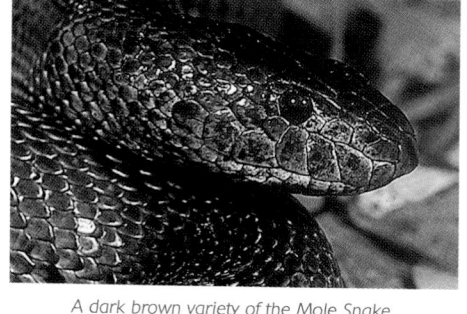

A dark brown variety of the Mole Snake.

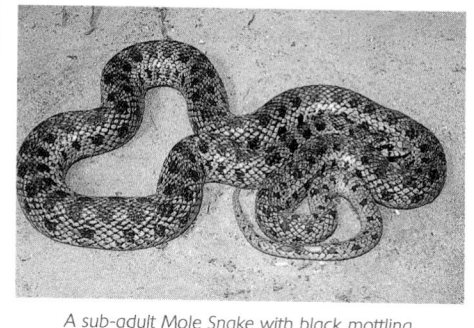

A sub-adult Mole Snake with black mottling.

Enemies

Predatory birds and snakes. Many individuals are killed by vehicles while basking on tarred roads.

Food and feeding

Adults feed on rats, moles, gerbils and other small land mammals. Birds and nestlings are taken, as are eggs – swallowed whole. Juveniles feed largely on lizards.

Reproduction

Viviparous, giving birth to an average 25-50 young or as many as 95 in late summer. The newborn snakes measure 20-31 cm in length.

Danger to man

Large adults may inflict a painful bite.

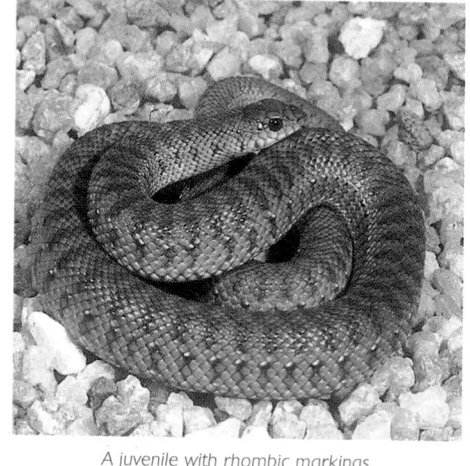

A juvenile with rhombic markings.

77

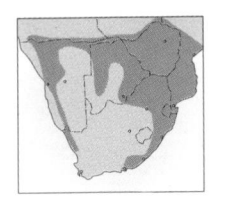

SPOTTED BUSH SNAKE

Philothamnus semivariegatus

HARMLESS

Other names
Variegated Bush
Snake (E)
Gespikkelde Bosslang (A)

Average 60-90 cm
Maximum 1,3 m

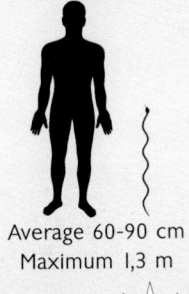
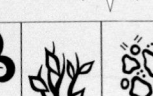
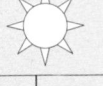
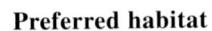

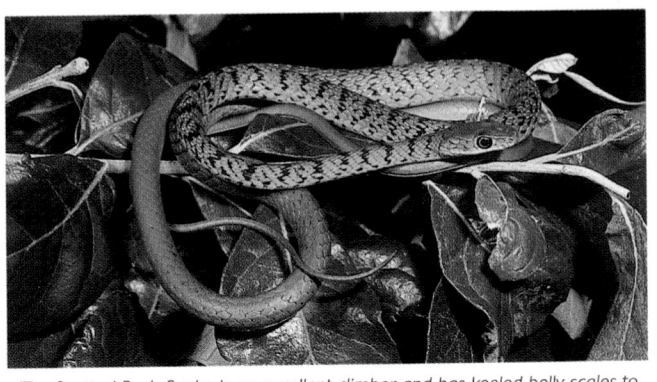

The Spotted Bush Snake is an excellent climber and has keeled belly scales to facilitate climbing up rough surfaces.

LOOK OUT FOR
- Usually has black speckles on the front half of the body.
- An expert climber.
- Often inhabits space between walls and corrugated roofing, especially in KwaZulu-Natal.
- Active during the day.

Preferred habitat
River banks, shrubs and bushes or rocky regions in Karoo, moist savanna and lowland forest.

Habits
A beautifully marked diurnal snake that moves gracefully or in short bursts if disturbed. It is an excellent climber and, with its keeled belly scales, can easily climb up the rough bark of a tree or even up face bricks. It often enters houses and outbuildings, especially those that have shrubs planted against the windows. When threatened, it may inflate its neck to expose the vivid blue skin between the scales. Like the Boomslang, it will

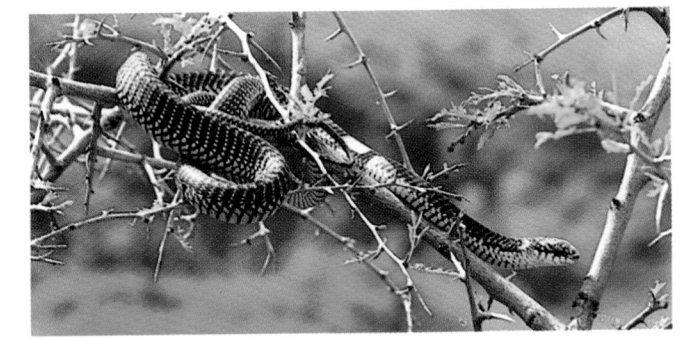

The Boomslang (above) is distinguished from the bush snake by its larger eyes.

raise its head off the ground and undulate the neck. The Spotted Bush Snake is very common throughout most of its range, often inhabiting the space between walls and corrugated roofs where it feeds on geckos. It soon moves off when disturbed and bites readily if handled.

Similar species

Because of its colour it is often mistaken for the Green Mamba and the Boomslang.

Enemies

Predatory birds and other snakes, especially the Twig Snake.

Food and feeding

Mainly lizards, especially geckos, and frogs (not toads).

Reproduction

Oviparous, laying 3-12 eggs (28-41 × 8-15 mm) in mid-summer. The young measure 23-30 cm.

Danger to man

None.

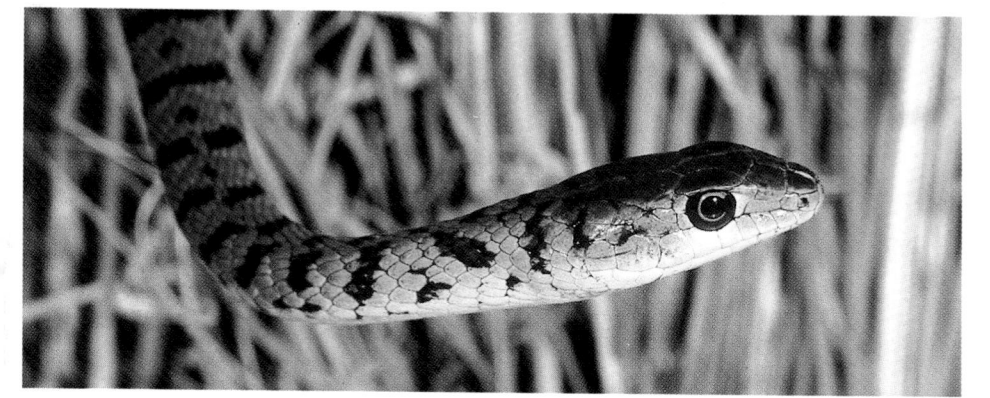

The Spotted Bush Snake is beautifully marked with characteristic black speckling on the front half of its body.

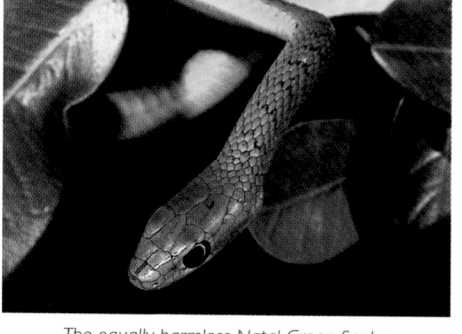

The equally harmless Natal Green Snake.

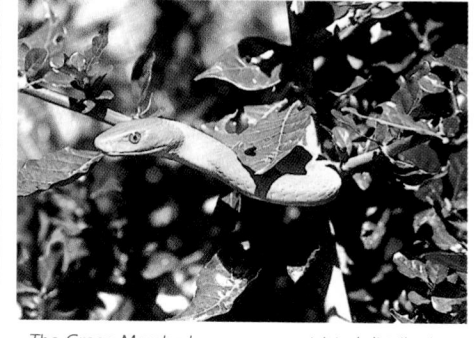

The Green Mamba has a more restricted distribution.

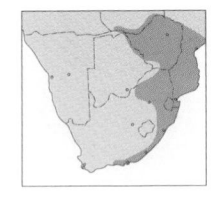

GREEN WATER SNAKE
Philothamnus hoplogaster

HARMLESS

Average 60 cm
Maximum nearly 1 m

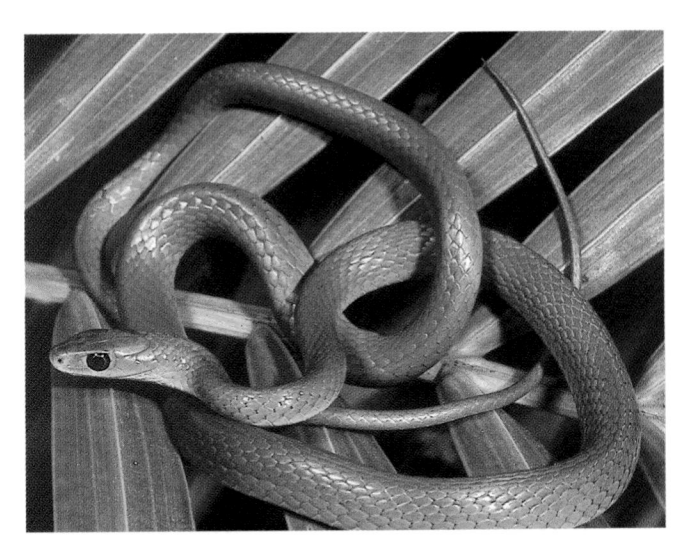

The harmless Green Water Snake (above) is sometimes confused with the venomous Green Mamba.

LOOK OUT FOR
- Usually bright emerald green above with a white or yellow belly.
- Very good swimmer.
- Active during the day.

Preferred habitat
Quite varied but common in moist savanna and lowland forest.

Habits
An active and alert diurnal snake that favours damp localities such as reed swamps, riverine thickets and flood plains of lakes and rivers. It is an excellent swimmer, but is also at home in shrubs and bushes.

Similar species
Because of its colour it is often mistaken for the Green Mamba. This snake is also easily confused with other harmless green snakes of the genus *Philothamnus*.

Enemies
Predatory birds and other snakes.

Food and feeding
Mainly frogs which may be captured in water and then carried back to land before they are swallowed. Fish and small lizards are also taken, while juveniles reportedly eat grasshoppers.

Reproduction
Oviparous, laying 3-8 elongate eggs (25-34 x 8-12 mm) in early summer. The young snakes measure 15–20 cm in length.

Danger to Man
None.

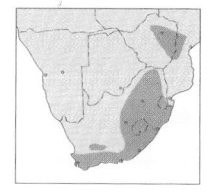

COMMON SLUG-EATER
Duberria lutrix

Other names
Gewone Slakvreter;
Tabakrolletjie (A)

Average 30–35 cm
Maximum 43 cm

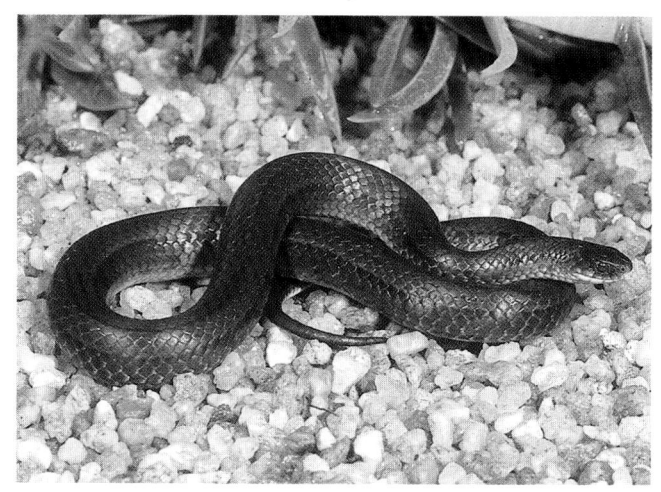

The Common Slug-eater favours damp localities where it has easy access to its slug and snail prey.

LOOK OUT FOR
- Has a small head hardly distinct from the rest of the body.
- Has powerful stink glands (which may be used in self-defence, especially when handled by man).
- May roll up into a tight spiral.
- Favours damp localities.

Preferred habitat
Largely a grassland inhabitant, but also found in moist savanna, lowland forest and fynbos.

Habits
A common, harmless species that favours damp localities where it preys on snails and slugs. It can be found beneath virtually any form of cover. It is a useful snake as it keeps down the snail population in gardens.

The slug-eater seldom attempts to bite, usually choosing to roll up tightly into a spiral with its head concealed, very much like a roll of tobacco, hence the Afrikaans name, *Tabakrolletjie*. It also has powerful stink glands which may be used in self-defence.

Similar species
May be confused with other small harmless snakes.

Enemies
Predatory birds and other snakes.

Food and feeding
Preys on slugs and snails. When consuming a snail, it will grasp the forepart of its prey and slowly pull the rest out of the shell.

Reproduction
Viviparous, giving birth in late summer to 6-22 young: 8-11 cm in length.

Danger to man
None.

81

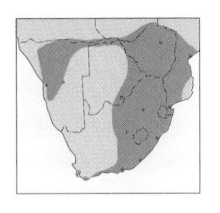

CAPE WOLF SNAKE
Lycophidion capense

Other names
Kaapse Wolfslang (A)

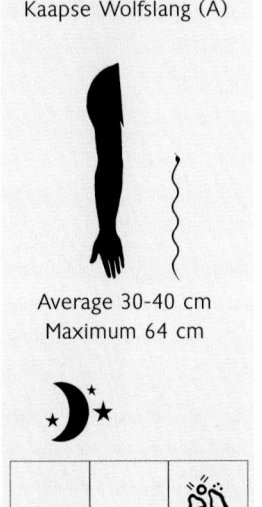

Average 30-40 cm
Maximum 64 cm

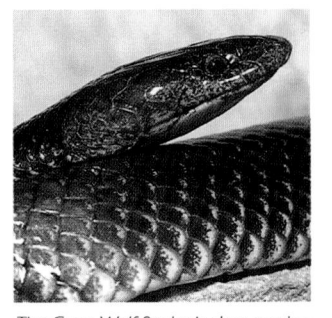
The Cape Wolf Snake

Preferred habitat
Lowland forest and fynbos to moist savanna, grassland and Karoo.

Habits
A terrestrial slow-moving constrictor that seldom attempts to bite. It is active at night when it hunts for lizards, especially skinks and geckos. It is fond of damp localities and is often found under stones, logs, piles of thatch grass, rubbish heaps or in deserted termite mounds. It has long recurved teeth on both the upper and lower jaws, which account for its common name. The teeth enable it to hold onto slippery prey.

Similar species
May be confused with a variety of other insignificant-looking snakes, including the venomous Stiletto Snake.

Enemies
Other snakes.

Food and feeding
Mainly lizards, including skinks and geckos.

The Cape Wolf Snake is slow moving and seldom attempts to bite.

Reproduction
Oviparous, laying from 3-9 eggs (22 × 10 mm) in early summer. The young measure 12 cm in length.

Danger to man
None.

LOOK OUT FOR
• Plain brown to black above with white-edged scales, which create a speckled effect.
• A flattened head, barely distinct from the rest of the body.
• Active at night.

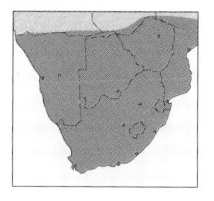

COMMON EGG-EATER

Dasypeltis scabra

HARMLESS

Other names
Rhombic Egg-eater (E)
Gewone Eiervreter (A)

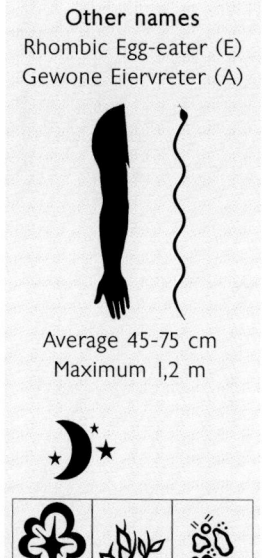

Average 45-75 cm
Maximum 1,2 m

LOOK OUT FOR
• Rhombic markings.
• One or more dark V-markings on the neck *behind* the head (the Night Adder, page24, has a V-marking on the head).
• The inside of the mouth is very dark.
• Active at night.

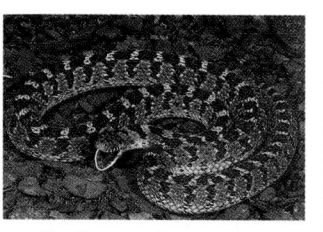

The Common Egg-eater in a defensive posture.

Preferred habitat
A common snake throughout most of southern Africa except the true desert and closed-canopy forest areas.

Habits
This snake is most abundant in dry thornveld and grasslands where it may be found in virtually any situation. It is nocturnal, spending most of the day hiding beneath rocks or under loose bark. It frequents disused termite mounds, especially in winter when it hibernates.

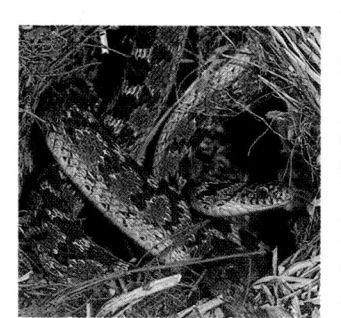

The Common Egg-eater

When agitated, it will coil and uncoil, allowing its roughly keeled scales on the sides to rub against each other, causing a hissing or rasping sound similar to the hiss of some adders. It will also strike out viciously with its mouth agape, exposing the dark lining of the mouth. As its diet consists largely of eggs, its teeth serve no purpose and are greatly reduced.

Similar species
The rhombic markings of this snake may cause confusion with the Night Adder in south-eastern Africa and with the Horned Adder in south-western Africa.

Enemies
Predatory birds and other snakes.

Food and feeding
Feeds on birds' eggs. An egg is taken into the virtually toothless mouth and passed onto the neck region. There it is cracked length-wise by a series of bony projections that are part of the vertebrae. Muscular contractions then crush the egg and the contents are swallowed. The crushed shell is regurgitated in a neat package.

Reproduction
Oviparous, laying 6-25 eggs (27-46 × 15-20 mm) in summer. The young measure 21-24 cm in length.

Danger to man
None.

BLIND SNAKES

Typhlops and *Rhinotyphlops* species

HARMLESS

Other names
Blindeslange (A)

Average 15-20 cm
Maximum 46 cm

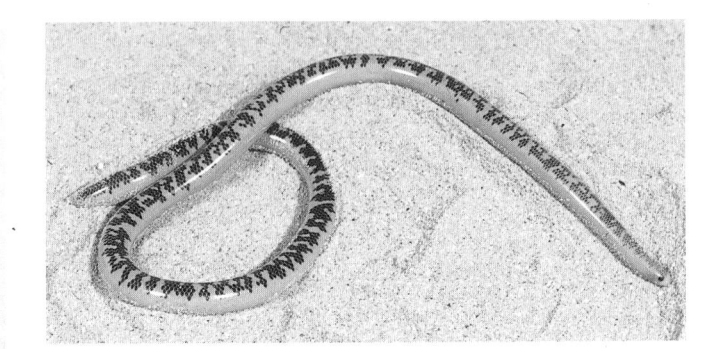

Above: A Blind Snake from Springbok, Namaqualand.
Below: A Blind Snake: note that the head is barely distinguishable from the body.

Preferred habitat

There are several different types of blind snakes; they inhabit a wide variety of habitats from Namib Desert to Karoo, grasslands, arid and moist savanna, lowland forest and fynbos.

Habits

Blind snakes are very primitive burrowing snakes that are well adapted to their underground existence. They have cylindrical bodies with highly polished scales, their heads are indistinct from the rest of the bodies and their eyes, which barely function, are greatly reduced. Most species are quite similar in appearance and colour.

Because of their underground existence, these snakes are seldom seen. Heavy rains may force them to the surface, while others are exposed during ploughing or digging operations. Otherwise they may be found under rocks or in termite mounds.

Similar species

May be confused with the venomous Stiletto Snake.

Enemies

Other snakes.

Food and feeding

Feeds on termites, their eggs and on other invertebrates.

Reproduction

Different species are either live-bearing or egg-laying. Only a few eggs are laid at a time.

Danger to man

None.

LOOK OUT FOR
- A cylindrical body with highly polished scales.
- A blunt head indistinct from the rest of the body.
- Eyes greatly reduced and barely visible.

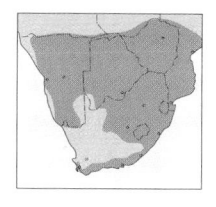

THREAD SNAKES

Leptotyphlops species

Other names
Erdslangetjie (A)

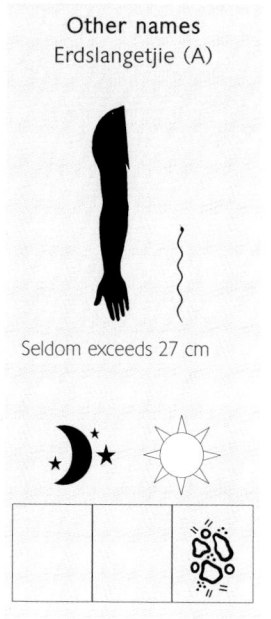

Seldom exceeds 27 cm

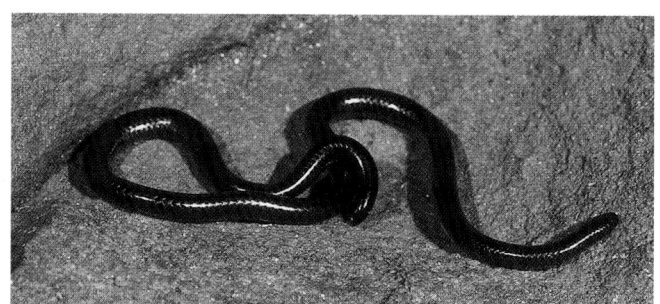

Primitive thread snakes are blind, their eyes reduced to dark spots. They have cylindrical bodies adapted for burrowing.

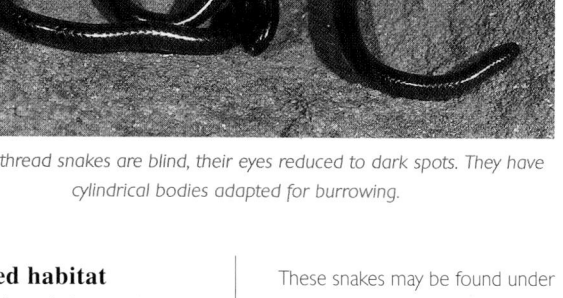

LOOK OUT FOR
- A snake that is very thin and small.
- A cylindrical body with highly polished scales.
- Head and tail cannot be distinguished from the rest of the body.

Preferred habitat
Thread snakes inhabit a wide variety of habitats, from fynbos to lowland forest, grassland, arid and moist savanna, and Karoo.

Habits
Small, thin, primitive snakes with no teeth in the upper jaw. They are burrowing snakes with a cylindrical body, a blunt head and highly polished scales. Thread snakes are blind, their eyes reduced to dark spots.

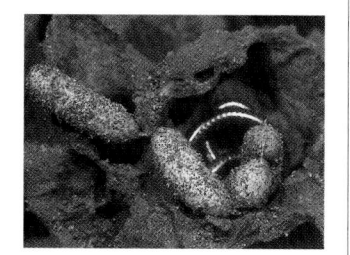

The rice-shaped eggs may be attached together like sausages.

These snakes may be found under rubble and in termite mounds, and many individuals are exposed during ploughing. Like the blind snakes, thread snakes are often flushed to the surface during heavy rains.

Enemies
Other snakes, spiders and scorpions.

Food and feeding
Actively feeds during the day and night. Prey includes ants, termites and other small invertebrates. Small prey is swallowed whole, while the abdomens of larger prey are sucked dry.

Reproduction
Oviparous, laying 1-7 elongate eggs in summer. The eggs are the size of rice grains and may be attached like sausages.

Danger to man
None.

85

GLOSSARY

Antivenom Used to combat the effects of snake venom, this is a crystallised serum produced from antibodies of animals infused with venom; capable of partially neutralising the venom's metabolism of the victim's tissue.

Aquatic Living in water.

Cytotoxic Poison that adversely affects tissue and cell formation. Predominant in adder venoms.

Diurnal Active mainly during the day.

Dorsal Pertaining to the upper surface of the body.

Elapid A rigidly front-fanged snake, belonging to the family Elapidae, e.g. cobras, Rinkhals, mambas and the Coral Snake.

Fang A large specialised tooth adapted for the injection of poison into prey.

Haemotoxic A substance poisonous to red blood cells, and adversely affecting the circulatory or blood system.

Hatchling A newborn reptile produced by an egg-laying species.

Keel A ridge on the scales of some snakes, e.g. the Boomslang.

Montane Pertaining to mountains.

Necrosis The death of cells (bone or soft tissue) in the body, usually within a localised area. Gangrene is necrosis plus infection.

Neurotoxic A poison that adversely affects neuromuscular function. Predominant in venoms of front-fanged snakes.

Nocturnal Active mainly at night.

Oviparous Egg-laying.

Recurved Descriptive of something that bends backwards.

Rhombic More or less diamond-shaped.

Riverine Pertaining to an area in or near rivers.

Terrestrial Ground-living.

Viviparous Pertaining to species which seemingly give birth to live young. In actual fact, the eggs hatch within the uterus of the female, or as the egg is being laid, or shortly after being laying. The eggs have a transparent membrane and lack the leathery white outer layer as seen in oviparous snakes.

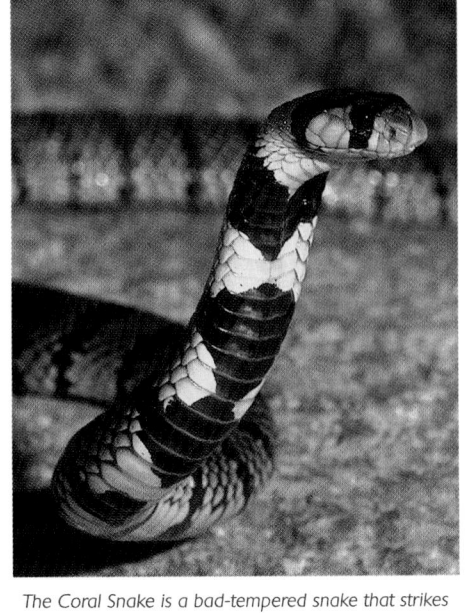

The Coral Snake is a bad-tempered snake that strikes readily if cornered.

FURTHER READING

Auerbach, R. 1987. *Reptiles and Amphibians of Botswana*. Mokwepa Consultants, Gaborone.

Branch, B. 1993. *Southern African Snakes and Other Reptiles – A Photographic Guide*. Struik Publishers.

Branch, B. 1998. *Field Guide to Snakes and Other Reptiles of Southern Africa*. Struik Publishers.

Marais, J. 1992. *A Complete Guide to Snakes of Southern Africa*. Southern Book Publishers.

Patterson, R. and Bannister, A. 1987. *South African Reptile Life*. Struik Publishers.

Pienaar, U. de V., Haacke, W.D. and Jacobson, N. 1983. *The Reptiles of the Kruger National Park*. National Parks Board, Pretoria.

Spawls, S. and Branch, W. R. 1995. *Dangerous Snakes of Africa*. Southern Book Publishers.

INDEX